D1764775

Oral Hygiene Methods

THE SCIENTIFIC WAY

Oral Hygiene Methods
The Scientific Way

1st edition

Printed in Sweden by Team Offset, Malmö

ISBN: 91-971823-3-8

This book can be ordered from:
OdontoScience
Klostergatan 1
211 47 Malmö
Sweden
fax no. +46-40-12 96 12

JAN EGELBERG

Oral Hygiene Methods

THE SCIENTIFIC WAY

Synopses of
Clinical Studies

OdontoScience

Contents

Preface

The purpose of this text is to present essential information on what is known about the efficacy of various oral hygiene methods. The information is presented in light of the need for scientific data to justify our recommendations to patients.

The book is a compilation of reviews of representative clinical studies. A uniform and condensed mode has been used to present the various trials. Following the presentation of the procedures and results, each review is accompanied with comments of my own. Concluding remarks relative to the overall findings and relative to the limitations of research for each topic are given at the end of each section.

The research reviews are not intended to be detailed. For a deeper and more critical understanding of the various studies presented, the reader should scrutinize the original research papers. This text may best serve its purpose when the need to do so is felt.

This book could prove useful for dentists and hygienists who want an update on research relating to oral hygiene methods. Students of dentistry and dental hygiene may also have an interest in the scientific basis for various recommendations to patients. Personally, I feel that there should be a definite need for this type of publication considering the multitude of marketing claims that we meet from commercial suppliers of various products. It is my aspiration that readers of this book will foster their desire to critically evaluate such claims.

Many readers of this text may prefer to 'sample' from the various sections, rather than reading the book from cover to cover. On the following page, I have made some suggestions that may facilitate reading and comprehension.

Jan Egelberg

Suggestions for reading

The following approach may be useful for reading this book:

1. Select topic/section from the table of contents.

2. Turn to the first page for that section and read the introduction.

3. Turn to the following page and review 'Studies Presented in this Section'.

4. Turn to the last page(s) of the section and read under 'Concluding Remarks'.

5. Read the individual study reviews.

Introductory remarks

Selection of studies

The selection of studies to be included for review in the various sections of this text has been a delicate task. An attempt has been made to include pertinent studies with typical results for the various topics. The ambition has been to select a limited number of studies, but also to provide representative results. Often, it has not been possible to meet this overall goal due to various reasons.

Sometimes, only a single or a very few studies have been published on a specific topic, and it has not been possible to establish any trend of results due to the limited information at hand. The available study/studies have been included, coupled with remarks about the limited information at hand.

Contradictory results of studies are not uncommon. In this situation, studies have been selected to illustrate this diversity.

More recent studies have been given preference in the selection process. For several topics, however, research activity has been low during recent years, and older studies have been included.

Obviously, the quality of the studies have been considered. It could be recognized that few of the available studies in the literature met all of the requirements of a 'perfect' study, but also that few studies had a quality which automatically excluded them for review.

With one exception, the content of this text is limited to oral hygiene procedures in adults. Although it would have been desirable, special groups like individuals with impaired dexterity and elderly people have not been included, since experimental studies do not seem to be available for such groups.

The topic of oral hygiene includes evaluation of commercially available products like toothbrushes, dentifrices and mouthwashes. Companies are trying to develop new products which are improvements over previous ones, and also over those of their competitors. The new products are usually evaluated in trials sponsored by the companies. Naturally, the companies are looking for results justifying claims of superiority. There are reasons to suspect that positive results for a given product have been published, while negative results may not have reached the literature. A reader reviewing the literature will notice that trials showing an advantage to a particular product typically has been sponsored by the manufacturer of this product. The possibility of a commercial influence on the available literature has been a concern in the selection process for studies to be included for review in this text. An attempt has been made to mitigate this problem by inclusion of trials representing the various products and commercial interests. It should be recognized, however, that for many products on the market there are no published research.

Study design

The vast majority of studies reviewed in this text are experimental trials. The effects of various oral hygiene methods have been compared in subjects belonging to different study groups, practicing the procedures to be evaluated. The reader of this book who is less familiar with designs and conduct of experimental trials might want to consult Appendix 2: Glossary of Experimental Designs (pages 279-291), prior to reading the main text.

Measurements for evaluation of results

The most commonly used methods to evaluate the effects of oral hygiene procedures are measurements of the amounts of dental plaque and the degree of gingivitis. The particular methods used vary among studies. Investigated sites in the dentition may be examined for presence or absence of plaque, gingivitis or bleeding on probing. Results are expressed as % positive or % negative sites relative to all examined sites. Alternatively, degrees of plaque accumulation and gingivitis may be recorded using plaque and gingival indices, where increasing levels of plaque and gingivitis are assigned increasing numerical scores, e.g. from 0 to 3. Details and comments relative to the most commonly used plaque and gingival indices are presented in Appendix 1: Commonly Used Plaque and Gingival Indices (pages 271-278).

Use of statistics

Results of statistical tests presented in the original publications have only occasionally been included or commented upon in this book. However, whenever the comments in the review of a particular study include terms like 'different from', 'higher than', 'lower than', etc., this corresponds to a statistically significant difference in the original publication. Often, the terms in the comments have been given a qualifier like 'somewhat', 'slightly' or 'little'. Also when these qualifiers are used, statistically significant differences are present. Terms like 'no difference' and 'similar' have been used when there are no statistically significant differences.

Descriptions of oral hygiene methods and aids

It is assumed that the reader of this text is familiar with most of the methods and devices for oral hygiene. Therefore, descriptions and illustrations of the various procedures and aids have not been included. Should a particular device that is reviewed and evaluated in this book be unknown, the reader is probably better guided by obtaining and physically examining this device than by looking at a photograph.

Effects on dental caries

Experimental studies of the effects of oral hygiene procedures on dental caries have not been included, since they have been considered beyond the scope of this text.

SECTION 1

Toothbrushing methods

During the 1970's several investigators compared the plaque removing efficacy of different methods of toothbrushing, e.g. Bass, Charters, circular, roll and scrub methods. In some of these studies in adults, the methods were compared after the subjects' abstinence of tooth cleaning during a number of days, followed by brushings performed by professionals. Other studies compared the techniques in 1-2 week trials with dental students brushing their own teeth. Results typically showed no or little difference between the various toothbrushing techniques. In addition, all methods proved inefficient for proximal surfaces, particularly in patients with open interdental areas. The consistency of these findings is probably the reason for the scarcity of continued research in this area. In order to provide an example of results on toothbrushing methods, this section includes a review of a study from 1984 comparing 4 methods of brushing using 2 different toothbrushes.

STUDY PRESENTED IN THIS SECTION

Authors	Page	Subjects	Toothbrushing methods evaluated	Observation interval
Bergenholtz et al. (1984)	15	Adults with healthy gingiva; with/without open interdental embrasures	Bass Roll Circular scrub Horizontal scrub	5 days

ARCHIVTECHNIK KUNZE

JOURNAL 24   JOURNAL 35   JOURNAL 67   report 24

ETP - 150 x 7,6 mm

Einstellung: |— 12,7 mm —| = 1/2"
Adjustment:

|— 7,6 —| |— 5,1 —| —| |— 6,95

BERGENHOLTZ ET AL. (1984) compared 4 methods of toothbrushing using 2 different toothbrushes.

Subjects and procedures:
* 24 subjects, 20-49 years of age, with healthy gingival conditions
    - 12 dental students/dentists without periodontal tissue breakdown
    - 12 patients, previously treated for periodontal disease, with open interdental embrasures

* Toothbrushing methods:
    - Bass
    - Roll
    - Circular scrub
    - Horizontal scrub

* Toothbrushes:
    - Soft brush with V-position of adjacent rows of tufts (Jordan)
    - Soft, multitufted, flat trim brush (Jordan)

* Dental prophylaxis provided at baseline (baseline plaque scores = 0)[†]

* Subjects instructed to abstain from all self-performed oral hygiene procedures for 5 days

* Once daily visits for brushings by 1 of 2 participating professionals, each treating 6 + 6 patients; total of 3 minutes for brushing all 4 quadrants

* Toothbrushing methods compared by quadrant allotment (quadrant design)[†]

* Toothbrushes compared during 2 repeated 5-day periods (cross-over design)[†]

* Presence/absence of plaque at the gingival margin scored for 4 teeth in each quadrant; 5 sites from both of buccal and lingual aspects of each tooth (mid-surface + 2 line angle locations + 2 proximal locations); details on tooth selection not given

* Analyses of plaque scores after 5 days for each of the 5 buccal and lingual sites (% of examined surfaces with plaque)

[†] See Appendix 2: Glossary of Experimental Designs (pages 279-291).

Results:

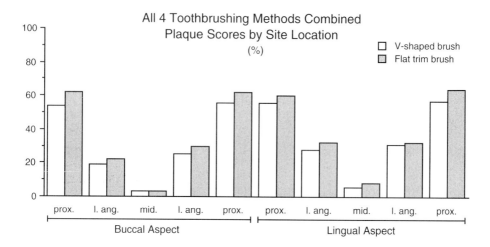

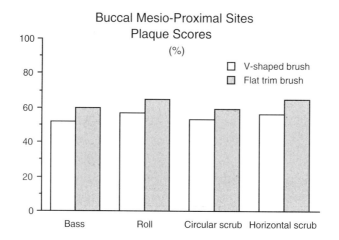

Comments:

- Plaque scores for all 4 toothbrushing methods combined showed little remaining plaque on the middle of buccal/lingual surfaces. For the line angle sites and for the proximal sites in particular, plaque removal was inefficient.

- Data on the comparisons of the 4 toothbrushing methods for buccal mesio-proximal surfaces failed to disclose any differences between the techniques. Although data were not given, the authors stated that the only positive finding was that the Bass method showed slightly - and statistically significantly - better plaque removal on some of the lingual aspects than the other methods.

- The results indicated some advantage to the V-shaped brush over the flat trim brush for proximal locations. Differences, however, were small relative to the levels of residual plaque. Around 55% of proximal sites continued to show plaque. (For additional studies on effects of various toothbrush designs, see Section 2: Manual Toothbrush Design, pages 21-43.)

- Surprisingly, the authors did not present separate data for the 2 subgroups of patients, but remarked that subjects with open embrasures showed more remaining plaque on proximal/interdental surfaces than subjects with intact dentition.

- There were no differences in results for the 2 professionals performing the brushings (data not shown here).

- Although not stated by the authors, it is to be assumed that the final plaque scores were taken around 24 hours after the last brushing?

- This study confirms the results of previous studies also observing little or no difference between brushing methods and their lack of effectiveness on proximal/interdental surfaces, particular in individuals with open dental embrasures (e.g. Hansen & Gjermo 1971, Gibson & Wade 1977, review by Frandsen 1986).

Toothbrushing methods

Concluding remarks

There seems to be little advantage to the use of a particular toothbrushing method for the purpose of removing dental plaque.

None of the toothbrushing techniques seems to be effective in eliminating proximal/interdental plaque.

Subjects and sites to be included in studies on toothbrushing effectiveness should be carefully selected with respect to presence of intact periodontal tissues (no reduction of papillary height) versus presence of open interdental embrasures (reduced papillary height). This will allow separate evaluations of the effects on *proximal* sites (i.e. the visible areas adjacent to intact papillae) and the effects on *interdental* sites (i.e. the areas underneath the contact point, exposed due to reduced papillary height).

Available studies on toothbrushing methods are short-term trials. Long-term evaluations do not seem to have been performed.

There seem to be no studies investigating to what extent patients continue to use a specific method of toothbrushing following instruction, or if they tend to revert to their previous habitual method.

Toothbrushing methods

References

Bergenholtz, A., Gustafsson, L.B., Segerlund, N., Hagberg, C. & Nygaard Östby, P. (1984) Role of brushing technique and toothbrush design in plaque removal. Scandinavian Journal of Dental Research 92, 344-351.

Frandsen, A. (1986) Mechanical oral hygiene practices. In *Dental Plaque Control Measures and Oral Hygiene Practices*, ed. Löe, H. & Kleinman, D.V., pp. 93-116, IRL Press, Oxford-Washington DC.

Gibson, J.A. & Wade, A.B. (1977) Plaque removal by the Bass and roll brushing techniques. Journal of Periodontology 48, 456-459.

Hansen, F. & Gjermo, P. (1971) The plaque-removing effect of four toothbrushing methods. Scandinavian Journal of Dental Research 80, 267-271.

SECTION 2

Manual toothbrush design

Studies in the past, comparing the effects of different toothbrush design, have observed little or no difference between various brushes available on the market. More recently, toothbrushes with novel designs have been introduced with claims of improved efficacy. Many studies on these brushes are 'single-use' tests, i.e. participating subjects have been brushing their teeth at a single time point with the brushes to be evaluated, often after abstaining from oral hygiene during a number of days prior to the tests. Other studies have compared the brushes following periods of use limited to a few weeks.

Although the single-use and short-term trials may be useful as pilot screening experiments, they need to be supplemented with studies of longer duration to allow an evaluation of continued and regular use of the brushes. Extended study periods will decrease the possibility of a 'novelty effect', i.e. reducing the probability that subjects using a new product may be more attentive and thorough using this product during an initial period of time than the use of a familiar product. Prolonged observation intervals will also allow the use of gingivitis scores in addition to plaque scores for assessment of results. Plaque scores are sensitive to the experimental situation, i.e. subjects may brush the teeth more carefully prior to the examination visits. Gingivitis scores are valuable supplements, since they may not be readily affected by occasional, improved toothbrushings.

Novel design brushes for adults have been evaluated in several single-use studies, but only in 4 longer-term trials. One single-use study is included in this section to provide an example, together with the 4 available longer-term trials.

STUDIES PRESENTED IN THIS SECTION

Authors	Page	Subjects	Brushes evaluated	Observation interval
Deasy et al. (1993)	23	Adults	Colgate Precision Reach Full Head Oral-B 40	Single-use
Reardon et al. (1993)	26	Adults with plaque and gingivitis	Crest Complete Oral-B P-35	3 months
Grossman et al. (1994)	29	Adults with plaque and gingivitis	Colgate Plus Colgate Precision Crest Complete Jordan Exact Oral-B Advantage Reach Advanced Design	2 months
Sharma et al. (1994)	33	Adults with plaque and gingivitis	Colgate Total New Improved Crest Complete Oral-B Advantage Reach Advanced Design	3 months
Yankell et al. (1996)	36	Adults with plaque and gingivitis	Dentrust Oral-B P-35	6 months

DEASY ET AL. (1993) compared 2 novel design toothbrushes to a regular flat trim brush in a single-use study.

Subjects and procedures:

* 75 employees of a medical/dental university, 20-64 years of age (details on any periodontal disease and on interdental papillary heights not provided)

* 3 study groups, matched for plaque scores (cross-over, rotating sequence design[†], total N=75):
    - Colgate Precision (presently marketed as Colgate Total)
    - Reach Full Head soft
    - Oral-B 40 (flat trim)

* Subjects asked to refrain from toothbrushing for 24 hours prior to tests

* On test days, plaque initially disclosed with a dye and recorded (prebrushing scores), followed by patients' unsupervised brushing for 1 minute with the assigned study brush using their habitual brushing method, followed by renewed plaque staining and recording (postbrushing scores)

* After 1 week of normal oral hygiene routine ('wash-out period'[†]), subjects returned for test using another toothbrush, repeated 1 week later to allow all subjects to use all 3 brushes

* Presence/absence of plaque scored at 9 buccal and 9 lingual sites of each tooth using disclosing dye and Rustogi/Navy index[††]

* Analyses of mean pre- and postbrushing plaque scores (% sites with plaque):
    - All sites (18 per tooth; 9 buccal + 9 lingual)
    - Gingival margin sites (6 per tooth; 3 buccal + 3 lingual)
    - Proximal sites (4 per tooth; 2 buccal + 2 lingual)

[†]   See Appendix 2: Glossary of Experimental Designs (pages 279-291).

[††] See Appendix 1: Commonly Used Plaque and Gingival Indices (pages 271-278).

Results:

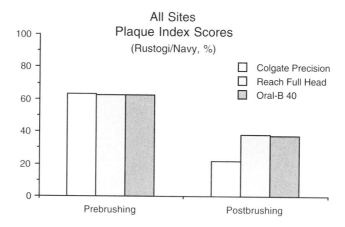

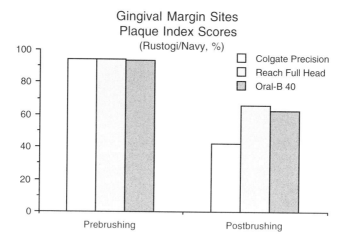

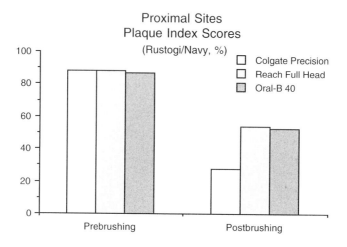

Comments:

- Plaque removal was observed to be more efficient following use of Colgate Precision than use of either Reach Full Head or Oral-B 40. This included scores for sites at the gingival margin only, for proximal sites only, and for all recorded sites in the dentition.

- The same 3 toothbrushes were compared in 2 other single-use studies using the same design and the same plaque index. Again, Colgate Precision was found more effective than the other brushes for sites at the gingival margin, for proximal sites, and for all sites (Sharma et al. 1992, Singh et al. 1992).

- Colgate Precision was compared to Crest Complete in 2 single-use studies also using the Rustogi/Navy plaque index, and was found more effective than this brush, also for all 3 groups of sites (Balanyk et al. 1993, Singh et al. 1993).

- Any use of dentifrice for the brushings in the above 5 studies can not be determined from the reports.

- In another single-use study using the Rustogi/Navy plaque index, an independent research group compared Colgate Precision to Aquafresh Flex, Crest Complete and Oral-B P-40 (using dentifrice), and found no differences in effectiveness for either gingival margin sites, proximal sites, or all sites (Claydon & Addy 1996).

- In still another single-use study, Reardon et al. (1993) compared Colgate Precision to Crest Complete and Oral-B P-35 using Turesky/Quigley-Hein plaque index, and did not observe any differences in plaque removal between the 3 toothbrushes (using dentifrice). Thus, results on effectiveness of Colgate Precision are contradictory.

- Single-use studies using professionals for the brushings and a quadrant design with different toothbrushing methods do not seem to be available (compare Bergenholtz et al. 1984, pages 15-17). This design may reduce the possibility of a novelty effect, and may also give information on the particular brushing conditions for the superiority, if any, of a particular toothbrush.

- The above single-use studies have not utilized baseline prophylaxes. This means that the subjects, upon entering each of the tests, may have a certain amount of adherent and stainable 'non-plaque' deposits that may be difficult to remove by toothbrushing. A design with baseline prophylaxis prior to each test period, followed by abstinence from tooth cleaning for a number of days, followed by pre- and postbrushing scores, could be a useful alternative.

REARDON ET AL. (1993) compared a novel design toothbrush to a regular flat trim brush in 2 similar 3-month studies.

Subjects and procedures:

* Adults with plaque and gingivitis at 2 different clinical trials institutes (details on any attachment loss/interdental papillary heights not provided)

* Study 1 test groups, matched for gingivitis and plaque (parallel design[†]; total N=140):
    - Crest Complete
    - Oral-B P-35 (flat trim)

* Study 2 test groups, matched for plaque and gingivitis (parallel design; total N=66):
    - Crest Complete
    - Oral-B P-35 (flat trim)

* Following baseline examination, subjects received prophylaxis (plaque scores = 0), the assigned toothbrush and a standard toothpaste, asked to brush with their habitual routine and to refrain from use of other toothpastes and mouthrinses

* Plaque scores at 6 locations of each tooth using disclosing dye and Turesky/ Quigley-Hein index (scores 0-5)[††]

* Gingivitis scores for buccal and lingual papillae and gingival margins of all teeth using Lobene index (scores 0-4)[††]

* 3 months of observation

* Analyses of mean plaque and gingivitis scores

[†]   See Appendix 2: Glossary of Experimental Designs (pages 279-291).
[††] See Appendix 1: Commonly Used Plaque and Gingival Indices (pages 271-278).

Results:

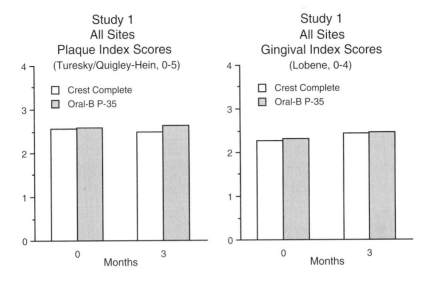

Study 1
All Sites
Plaque Index Scores
(Turesky/Quigley-Hein, 0-5)

☐ Crest Complete
▨ Oral-B P-35

Months

Study 1
All Sites
Gingival Index Scores
(Lobene, 0-4)

☐ Crest Complete
▨ Oral-B P-35

Months

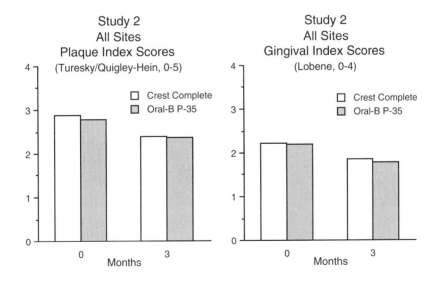

Study 2
All Sites
Plaque Index Scores
(Turesky/Quigley-Hein, 0-5)

☐ Crest Complete
▨ Oral-B P-35

Months

Study 2
All Sites
Gingival Index Scores
(Lobene, 0-4)

☐ Crest Complete
▨ Oral-B P-35

Months

Comments:

- Both studies demonstrated lack of difference between the 2 brushes.

- In Study 1, mean plaque scores after 3 months corresponded to the baseline scores prior to prophylaxis. The gingivitis scores also concurred with baseline levels.

- In Study 2, both plaque and gingivitis levels were lower after 3 months than at baseline. The subjects of this study may have improved their toothbrushing as an effect of being included in a trial (participation effect). However, it can not be excluded that these seeming changes, at least in part, can be explained by 'examiner drift', a phenomenon that may afflict parallel design studies. Assuming that all subjects of the study were carried through the experiment simultaneously, the examiner recorded baseline and final scores around 3 months apart, cognisant of visit sequence. Using subjective scoring systems like plaque and gingival indices, an examiner may change the implementation of the scoring system somewhat over time. Expectation of some improvement may cause an examiner drift in that direction.

- Results of plaque and gingival indices for proximal sites were presented separately (data not shown here). Although these scores were somewhat higher than the corresponding scores for all recorded sites around the teeth, results paralleled the findings for all sites in both studies.

- Mean 3-month plaque scores for all recorded sites in the dentition for the 2 studies ranged between 2.4-2.6. This means that overall, the participating subjects continued to show a band of plaque along the gingival margin. Mean 3-month gingivitis scores ranged between 1.8-2.4. This translates into an overall persistence of mild gingivitis around the teeth (see Appendix 1: Commonly Used Plaque and Gingival Indices; Turesky/Quigley-Hein plaque index, page 271; Lobene gingival index, page 275).

GROSSMAN ET AL. (1994), in 2 similar studies, evaluated a total of 6 different toothbrushes over periods of 2 months.

Subjects and procedures:
* Adults with plaque and gingivitis, 18-63 years of age, but "without evidence of periodontitis" (= intact papillary heights?)

* Study 1 test groups (parallel design; total N=109):
  - Colgate Precision (presently Colgate Total)
  - Crest Complete
  - Oral-B Advantage

* Study 2 test groups (parallel design; total N=121):
  - Colgate Plus (flat trim)
  - Jordan Exact
  - Oral-B Advantage
  - Reach Advanced Design

* After baseline examination, subjects received prophylaxis (plaque scores = 0), the assigned toothbrush and a standard toothpaste, asked to brush twice daily and to refrain from use of other oral hygiene aids

* Instructions not to brush for 24 hours before baseline and follow-up visits

* Plaque scores at 6 locations of each tooth using disclosing dye and Turesky/ Quigley-Hein index (scores 0-5)

* Gingivitis scores for buccal and lingual papillae and gingival margins of all teeth using Lobene index (scores 0-4)

* 2 months of observation

* Analyses of mean plaque and gingivitis scores

Results:

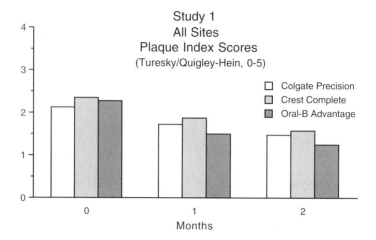

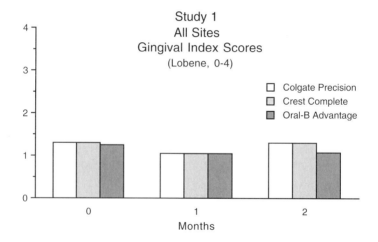

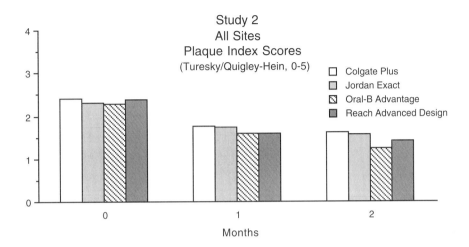

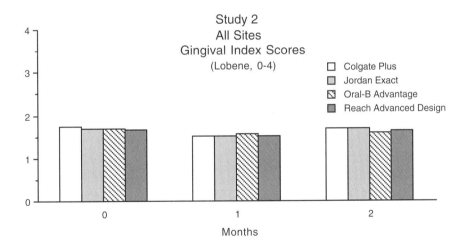

Comments:

- Mean plaque scores after 1 and 2 months for both studies appeared improved as compared to scores taken at baseline prior to prophylaxis. Gingivitis scores, however, remained unchanged.

- The possibility of some examiner drift needs to be considered for the interpretation of the plaque score results.

- The combined results of plaque and gingivitis scores indicate a slight benefit to Oral-B Advantage compared to the other brushes (reported to reach statistical significance for some of the comparisons). However, considering that the subjects were recruited on the basis of having plaque and gingivitis above a certain level, and the questionable changes over time, any benefit to Oral-B Advantage probably has little or no clinical significance.

- The authors also presented separate data for proximal sites (data not shown here). On average, proximal plaque and gingivitis scores were higher than corresponding scores for all recorded sites. Results for both studies, however, demonstrated similar trends as for all surfaces combined.

- Studies on toothbrushing often use recordings of '24-hour plaque' at the follow-up examinations, similar to the above study. This is believed to reduce the impact of extra cleaning efforts by the patients prior to the examinations, although this does not seem to have been supported by research findings. In other studies using 24-hour plaque, after an initial recording at the examination visit, subjects have been asked to brush their teeth with the assigned brush, followed by a repeated recording. Thus, at each examination, both pre-brushing and postbrushing scores are obtained and presented. This method of supplementation of the plaque data was not utilized in the study reviewed here.

SHARMA ET AL. (1994) compared 4 different toothbrushes over 3 months.

Subjects and procedures:

* 193 adults, 18-64 years of age, with plaque and gingivitis (details on any attachment loss/interdental papillary heights not provided)

* 4 study groups, matched for plaque and gingivitis (parallel design):
    - Colgate Total (formerly Colgate Precision) (N=50)
    - New Improved Crest Complete (N=49)
    - Oral-B Advantage (N=47)
    - Reach Advanced Design (N=47)

* Subjects given prophylaxis and returned for baseline examination after 48 hours of no oral hygiene, followed by provision of the assigned toothbrush and a regular toothpaste, and asked to brush twice daily

* Instructions not to brush during 24 hours before each follow-up visit

* Plaque scores for 9 buccal and 9 lingual locations of each tooth using disclosing dye and Rustogi/Navy index (%, based upon presence/absence in 18 locations per tooth)

* Gingivitis scores for buccal and lingual papillae and gingival margins of all teeth using Lobene index (scores 0-4)

* 12 weeks of observation

* Analyses of mean plaque and gingivitis scores

Results:

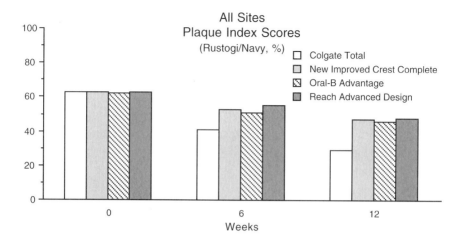

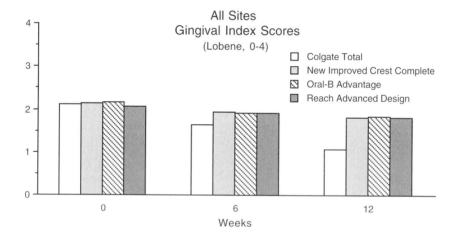

Comments:

- It is unclear why plaque scores at baseline were taken 48 hours after prophy-laxis and why scores at 6 and 12 weeks were obtained 24 hours after brush-ing. References to baseline are complicated by this inconsistency. Never-theless, the overall results of plaque and gingivitis scores show an advantage to Colgate Total over the other brushes.

- The benefits for Colgate Total included a benefit over Oral-B Advantage. These results are contradictory to the results by Grossman et al. (1994), who found a slight benefit to Oral-B Advantage over Colgate Total (see pages 29-32). Additional and independent study is needed to clarify this discrepancy.

- The opportunity to supplement the plaque data with postbrushing scores of the 24-hour plaque at the 6- and 12-week examinations was not exercised.

- The Rustogi/Navy plaque index was developed by the same research group as that for the above study to allow for a more sensitive evaluation of different gingival and proximal locations of buccal and lingual tooth surfaces (Rustogi et al. 1992, compare study by Deasy et al. 1993, pages 23-25). The authors did not utilize the opportunity to present findings for these specific surface loca-tions.

YANKELL ET AL. (1996) compared a triple-headed toothbrush to a conventional brush over 6 months.

Subjects and procedures:

* Adults, 18-60 years of age, with plaque and gingivitis (details on any attachment loss/interdental papillary heights not provided)

* Study groups (parallel design):
    - Dentrust (3-headed, 'monorail' brush to enable simultaneous cleaning of buccal, lingual and occlusal surfaces) (N=48)
    - Oral-B P-35 (flat trim) (N=45)

* Baseline examination 12-14 hours after last toothbrushing ('overnight plaque'), followed by monitored 1-min brushing with assigned brush, followed by repeated examination

* No baseline prophylaxis

* Pre- and postbrushing recordings of 'overnight plaque' repeated after 3 and 6 months of daily use of assigned brush

* Plaque scores at 6 locations of each tooth using disclosing dye and Turesky/Quigley-Hein index (scores 0-5)

* Gingivitis scores for buccal and lingual papillae and gingival margins of all teeth using Lobene index (scores 0-4)

* 6 months of observation

* Analyses of mean plaque and gingivitis scores for buccal and lingual aspects of the teeth

Results:

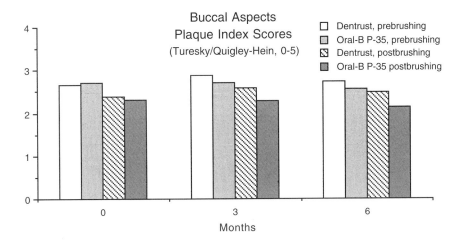

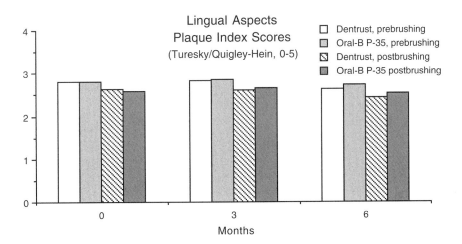

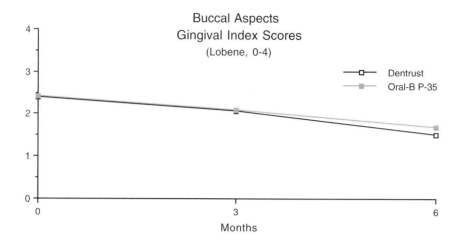

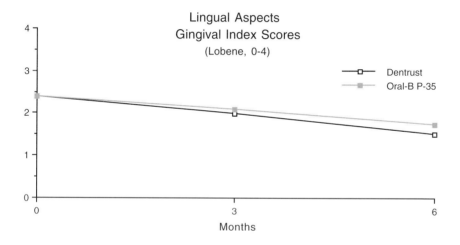

Comments:

- Mean plaque scores remained comparatively high throughout the study, and similar for both toothbrush groups.

- Plaque removal following the 1-min brushings at the examination intervals was limited for both brushes. For buccal aspects, plaque removal tended to be somewhat better for the conventional brush.

- The authors did not comment upon their use of 1 minute only for the brushings at the examinations.

- Mean gingivitis levels were reduced during the 6 months of study, but remained relatively high. Little difference was noted between brushes, although the difference in favor of Dentrust over the conventional brush reached statistical significance for the lingual aspects.

- The improvements of the gingivitis scores are somewhat unexpected in view of the unchanged plaque scores over the 6 months of study. A result of examiner drift?

- Separate data for proximal sites would have been of interest.

- Different brands of double-headed brushes have been compared to conventional toothbrushes by Bastiaan (1984), Gibson et al. (1988) and Agerholm (1991). Slightly better plaque removal for lingual surfaces has been noted for the double-headed brushes.

Manual toothbrush design

Concluding remarks

Results of several single-use studies suggest that Colgate Total is more effective in removing plaque than other toothbrushes. These results, however, were not confirmed in other single-use studies, observing no difference between Colgate Total and other tested brushes.

Among the longer-term studies, a noticeable benefit to Colgate Total was observed by Sharma et al. (1994) (pages 33-35). This was contradicted by the findings of Grossman et al. (1993) (pages 29-32).

In the longer-term trials, the overall impact on plaque and gingivitis levels in the participating subjects during the course of the studies is strikingly limited. Plaque and gingivitis scores often remain similar to the baseline scores in spite of the fact that the subjects are enrolled in a trial, given new design toothbrushes, and asked to return for repeated examinations.

The participants of the trials have typically been instructed to continue their habitual method of toothbrushing. The limited overall impact on plaque and gingivitis levels during the course of the trials suggests that these habitual brushing routines are inadequate. It may not be realistic to expect that any particular toothbrush design should be able to compensate for this inadequacy.

Subjects included in the toothbrush studies have been selected on the basis of presence of plaque and gingivitis. Details on presence of any attachment loss/reduced papillary heights have generally not been presented. As mentioned before, subjects and sites to be included in studies on toothbrushing effectiveness ought to be carefully selected with respect to presence of intact periodontal tissues (no reduction of papillary height) versus presence of open interdental embrasures (reduced papillary height).

There is nowadays evidence that smokers respond to dental plaque with a lower degree of gingivitis than the response in nonsmokers. Studies evaluating the effects of oral hygiene methods on gingivitis, therefore, should have study groups matched for proportions of smokers/nonsmokers. This does not seem to have been considered in the available trials on manual toothbrush design (and neither in studies on other oral hygiene methods!). Trials using study groups matched for both plaque and gingivitis, however, may indirectly achieve this effect.

Plaque and gingivitis data in studies on oral hygiene methods are commonly presented as means for all tooth sites combined. More emphasis on data analysis for proximal sites alone would be preferable. From a clinical perspective, data on % plaque-free and % gingivitis-free proximal sites would seem to the most meaningful way of evaluating effects of different oral hygiene methods.

Regrettably, the incidence of gingival abrasion following use of the various toothbrushes was not systematically studied in any of the available long-term trials.

Manual toothbrush design

References

Agerholm, D.M. (1991) A clinical trial to evaluate plaque removal with a double-headed toothbrush. British Dental Journal 170, 411-413.

Balanyk, T.E., Sharma, N.C. & Galustians, J. (1993) A clinical study of comparative plaque removal performance of two manual toothbrushes. Journal of Clinical Dentistry, 4, suppl. D, D8-D12.

Bastiaan, R.J. (1984) Comparison of the clinical effectiveness of a single and double headed toothbrush. Journal of Clinical Periodontology 11, 331-339.

Bergenholtz, A., Gustafsson, L.B., Segerlund, N., Hagberg, C. & Nygaard Östby, P. (1984) Role of brushing technique and toothbrush design in plaque removal. Scandinavian Journal of Dental Research 92, 344-351.

Claydon, N. & Addy, M. (1996) Comparative single-use plaque removal by toothbrushes of different design. Journal of Clinical Periodontology 23, 1112-1116.

Deasy, M.J., Singh, S.M., Kemp, J.H., Curtis, J.P., Rustogi, K.N. & Fung, K. (1993) A clinical comparison of plaque removal performance of three manual toothbrushes. Journal of Clinical Dentistry, 4, suppl. D, D17-D21.

Gibson, J.A. & Wade, A.B. (1977) Plaque removal by the Bass and roll brushing techniques. Journal of Periodontology 48, 456-459.

Gibson, M.T., Joyston-Bechal, S. & Smales, F.C. (1988) Clinical evaluation of plaque removal with a double-headed toothbrush. Journal of Clinical Periodontology 15, 94-98.

Grossman, E., Dembling, W. & Walley, D.R. (1994) Two long-term clinical studies comparing the plaque removal and gingivitis reduction efficacy of the Oral-B Advantage Plaque Remover to five manual toothbrushes. Journal of Clinical Dentistry 5, 46-53.

Hansen, F. & Gjermo, P. (1971) The plaque-removing effect of four toothbrushing methods. Scandinavian Journal of Dental Research 80, 267-271.

Reardon, R.C., Cronin, M., Balbo, F., Schiff, T., Menaker, L., Weatherford III, T.W., Walley, D. & Vidra, J. (1993) Four clinical studies comparing the efficacy of flat-trim and multi-level trim commercial toothbrushes. Journal of Clinical Dentistry 4, 101-105.

Rustogi, K.N., Curtis, J.P., Volpe, A.R., Kemp, J.H., McCool, J.J. & Korn, L.R. (1992) Refinement of the modified navy plaque index to increase the plaque scoring efficiency in gumline and interproximal tooth areas. Journal of Clinical Dentistry 3, suppl. C, C9-C12.

Sharma, N.C., Galustians, J., Rustogi, K.N., McCool, J.J., Petrone, M., Volpe, A.R., Korn, L.R. & Petrone, D. (1992) Comparative plaque removal efficacy of three toothbrushes in two independent clinical studies. Journal of Clinical Dentistry, 3, suppl. C, C13-C20.

Sharma, N.C., Galustians, J., McCool, J.J., Rustogi, K.N. & Volpe, A.R. (1994) The clinical effects on plaque and gingivitis over three-month's use of four complex-design manual toothbrushes. Journal of Clinical Dentistry 5, 114-118.

Singh, S.M. & Deasy, M.J. (1993) Clinical plaque removal performance of two manual toothbrushes. Journal of Clinical Dentistry, 4, suppl. D, D13-D16.

Singh, S.M., Rustogi, K.N., McCool, J.J., Petrone, M., Volpe, A.R., Korn, L.R. & Petrone, D. (1992) Comparative plaque removal efficacy of three toothbrushes in two independent clinical studies. Journal of Clinical Dentistry, 3, suppl. C, C21-C28.

Yankell, S.L., Emling, R.C. & Perez, B. (1996) A six-month clinical evaluation of the Dentrust toothbrush. Journal of Clinical Dentistry 7, 106-109.

Interdental cleaning

Interdental plaque control may be practiced with dental floss, woodsticks, single-tufted (end-tufted) brushes and interdental brushes. Dental floss of different types are available. To facilitate the use of floss, various types of flossing aids have been introduced. The design of woodsticks, single-tufted brushes and interdental brushes also vary among manufacturers. An electrically powered interdental cleaner has recently been marketed.

For this section, 6 studies are reviewed to provide examples of studies on the efficacy of various interdental aids in adults.

STUDIES PRESENTED IN THIS SECTION

CIANCIO ET AL. (1992) compared use of waxed nylon floss to expanded poly-tetrafluoroethylene ('teflon') floss.

Subjects and procedures:

* 57 subjects, 18-63 years of age, showing interdental plaque and gingivitis

* Details on interdental papillary height/open embrasures not presented

* Pre-experimental flossing habits not reported

* 2 study groups (parallel design):
    - Manual toothbrush + waxed nylon floss (N=30)
    - Manual toothbrush + expanded polytetrafluoroethylene (ePTFE) floss (Glide Floss) (N=27)

* Following baseline recordings, subjects instructed to supplement their regular toothbrushing with flossing once daily using assigned floss; toothbrush and dentifrice also provided

* No baseline prophylaxis

* Plaque scores at 6 locations of each tooth using disclosing dye and Turesky/Quigley-Hein index (scores 0-5)

* Presence/absence of interdental bleeding following 4 x interdental insertion and papillary depressing with a triangular woodstick (Eastman interdental bleeding index, % bleeding interdental areas[†])

* 5 weeks of observation

* Analyses of mean plaque scores for all surfaces and % bleeding interdental areas

† See Appendix 1: Commonly Used Plaque and Gingival Indices (pages 271-278).

Results:

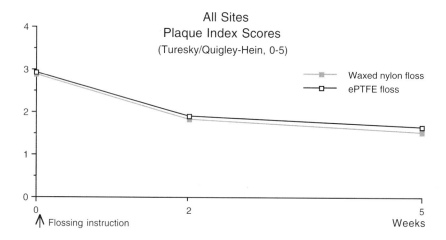

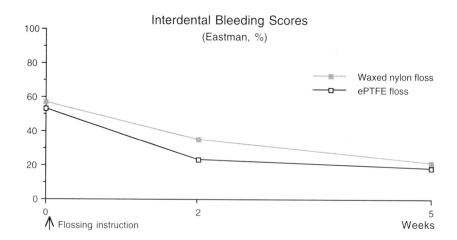

Comments:

- Mean plaque scores for all surfaces were reduced and to the same degree following use of both types of flosses. Plaque scores limited to proximal surfaces were not presented.

- At baseline, around 55% of all interdental areas in the dentition showed bleeding. The bleeding scores were similarly reduced following both flosses.

- The results of this study suggest that use of dental floss will reduce plaque levels and improve inderdental gingival health. Presumably, the participating subjects had previously not used dental floss on a regular basis, although this was not mentioned by the authors.

- A 3rd study group - use of toothbrush alone - would have been desirable. The results for this group would show if toothbrushing alone would affect the scores under the conditions of the trial (participation effect). Comparison of the 2 interdental cleaning groups to a toothbrushing only group would also control for any examiner drift.

- Other types of dental floss have also been compared. Typically, little or no differences in effectiveness have been found between various floss types. Thus, unwaxed and waxed nylon floss, unwaxed and waxed silk floss, Special Floss and SuperFloss were compared by Bergenholtz and Brithon (1980); unwaxed floss and SuperFloss by Stevens (1980) and by Abelson et al. (1981); unwaxed and waxed floss by Lamberts et al. (1982); unwaxed, waxed and mint-flavored floss by Lobene et al. (1982); waxed floss and SuperFloss by Wong & Wade (1985); unwaxed dental floss and SuperFloss by Spindel & Person (1987); waxed and unwaxed floss and dental tape by Graves et al. (1989); and waxed floss, dental tape and SuperFloss by Ong (1990).

CARTER-HANSON ET AL. (1996) compared finger flossing to use of a floss aid.

Subjects and procedures:

* 29 subjects, 22-68 years of age, previously not using dental floss regularly, showing interdental plaque and gingivitis, without having advanced periodontitis, and with no manual dexterity limitations

* Details on interdental papillary height/open embrasures not presented

* 2 study periods of 30 days each, separated by 14 days (cross-over design):
    - Manual toothbrush + unwaxed dental floss
    - Manual toothbrush + disposable floss aid (Quik Floss)

* Following baseline recordings, subjects instructed to supplement their regular toothbrushing with flossing using assigned regimen, once daily for 1st 30-day period (floss and toothbrush provided)

* After an interval of 14 days with no interdental cleaning ('wash-out period'), new 'baseline' recordings and instruction with the other flossing regimen

* No baseline prophylaxes

* Plaque scores at 4 proximal sites of each tooth (2 from buccal + 2 from lingual) using disclosing dye and Turesky/Quigley-Hein index (scores 0-5)

* Presence/absence of interdental bleeding after 4 x interdental insertion and papillary depressing with a triangular woodstick (Eastman interdental bleeding index, % bleeding interdental areas)

* Analyses of mean proximal plaque scores and % bleeding interdental areas

Results:

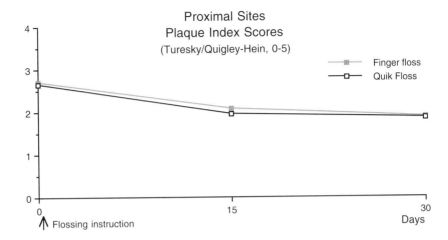

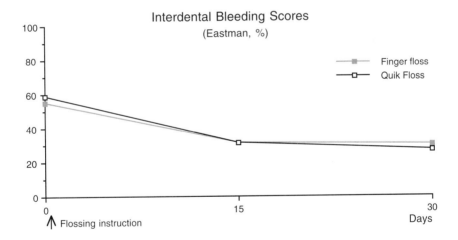

Comments:

- Proximal plaque scores were reduced and to the same extent following both flossing methods.

- Interdental bleeding scores were also equally reduced following both flossing methods. The bleeding score results, however, are confounded by the fact that the 2nd 30-day period most likely was affected by the 1st 30-day period, i.e. the baseline bleeding scores at the start of the 2nd 30-day period was presumably reduced compared to baseline scores for the 1st 30-day period. This may not have invalidated the comparison between the 2 interdental cleaning regimens, since one half of subjects used different aids during the 2 study periods. However, use of a cross-over study design seems questionable for evaluation of gingivitis.

- Similar to the results of Ciancio et al. (1992) (pages 47-49), this study suggests that introduction of flossing in subjects who previously may not have used floss on a regular basis will reduce plaque levels and improve inderdental gingival health. Improvements of plaque and gingivitis scores in both of these studies, however, levelled off without reaching optimal plaque control and gingival health.

- A 3rd study group - use of manual toothbrush alone - would have been desirable to control for any participation effect and examiner drift.

- The authors also evaluated the buccal and lingual tissues for gingival lacerations, but observed no significant trauma for either floss groups.

- Other floss holding devices have also been evaluated (EZ Denta-Flosser: Barton & Diamond 1980; Dr Flosser: Kleber & Putt 1988; Flosser: Spolsky et al. 1993; Floss Plus: Pucher et al. 1995). All of these studies have observed no difference between use of floss aid and finger flossing.

CRONIN & DEMBLING (1996) compared finger flossing to the use of an electrically powered interdental cleaner with rotating filaments.

Subjects and procedures:

* 48 subjects, 18-65 years of age, previously not using dental floss regularly, showing interdental plaque and gingivitis

* Subjects with "advanced periodontitis", and with "wide embrasure areas or gingival recession" not included

* 2 study groups (parallel design):
    - Manual toothbrush + waxed dental floss (N=24)
    - Manual toothbrush + Braun Oral-B Interclean (N=24)

* Following baseline recordings, subjects received prophylaxis (plaque scores = 0) and instruction in modified Bass toothbrushing (twice daily) and interdental cleaning with assigned method (once daily); interdental aids, toothbrush and dentifrice provided

* Subjects instructed to refrain from tooth cleaning 12-16 hours prior to examinations to allow overnight plaque formation

* Plaque scores at 4 proximal locations of each tooth using disclosing dye and Benson/Quigley-Hein index (scores 0-5)

* Presence/absence of bleeding on probing at 4 proximal locations of each tooth (% bleeding sites)

* 6 weeks of observation

* Analyses of mean proximal plaque and bleeding scores

Results:

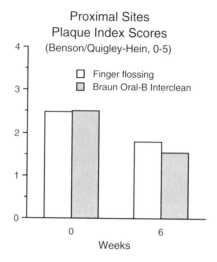

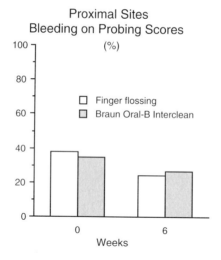

Comments:

- Plaque scores after 6 weeks were lower than the baseline scores prior to pro-phylaxis, and similar following use of both types of interdental cleaning meth-ods.

- Proximal bleeding scores were also similarly reduced following both cleaning methods. The reductions could be an effect of the introduction of interdental cleaning in the participating subjects, but possibly also due to the baseline prophylaxis and to a participation effect. A 3rd study group - toothbrushing alone - would have controlled for participation effect and examiner drift. A split-mouth design in addition to this, using prophylaxis in only half of the dentition would have controlled for the effect of the prophylaxis, and provided a comparison of the effects of interdental cleaning with and without prior pro-phylaxis.

- A 2nd set of plaque scores obtained at the 6-week examination after an addi-tional cleaning would have been of interest as a supplement to the records of the overnight plaque (pre- and postcleaning scores).

- The authors stated that "no adverse events or clinically significant occurrences were reported or observed during the study".

- Gordon et al. (1996), in an 1-month trial of similar design as the study reviewed above, also observed comparable results following finger flossing and use of Braun Oral-B Interclean (rotating filaments). They also reported "no evidence of significant soft tissue damage".

- More detailed studies and with longer duration may be required to evaluate any injurious effects of the electric interdental cleaner.

- The Braun Oral-B Interclean is also provided with a rubber tip attachment to be used for larger interdental spaces. This device was also found to reduce proximal plaque and bleeding scores to a similar extent as finger flossing in an 1-month trial (Cronin et al. 1997). Again and regrettably, this study used baseline prophylaxis and did not include a control group with toothbrushing alone.

BARTON & ABELSON (1987) studied the efficacy of triangular woodsticks in reducing interdental gingivitis.

Subjects and procedures:
* 77 subjects, 21 years and older, previously not using interdental cleaning aids, showing interdental gingivitis

* Details on interdental papillary height/open embrasures not presented

* 2 study groups (parallel design):
    - Manual toothbrush alone (N=39)
    - Manual toothbrush + balsawood triangular stick (Stim-U-Dent) (N=38)

* Following baseline recordings, subjects were provided a toothbrush and instructed to continue their regular toothbrushing, twice daily during 2 weeks, and to refrain from using additional oral hygiene aids

* No baseline prophylaxis

* Following repeated recordings after 2 weeks, subjects assigned toothbrush alone asked to continue this activity, and subjects assigned triangular wood-sticks instructed in their use and to be used in conjunction with toothbrushing

* Presence/absence of interdental bleeding following 4 x interdental insertion and papillary depressing with a triangular woodstick (Eastman interdental bleeding index, % bleeding interdental areas)

* 4 weeks of observation (between week 2 and week 6)

* Analyses of % bleeding interdental areas

Results:

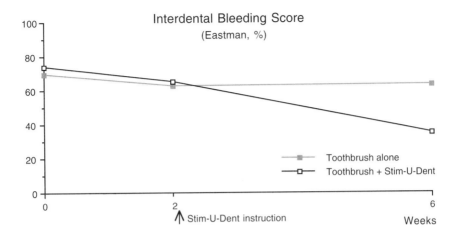

Comments:
- At baseline, 70-75% of all interdental areas in the dentition showed bleeding. Compared to continued use of toothbrush alone, the introduction of triangular woodsticks at 2 weeks resulted in reduced interdental bleeding.

- Plaque scores were not recorded.

- A 3rd study group - use of dental floss - would have been of interest, as would continuation of the study beyond 6 weeks of observation.

WOLFFE (1976) evaluated plaque removal efficacy of dental floss, woodsticks and a single-tufted brush in open interdental embrasures.

Subjects and procedures:

* 35 patients, 19-54 years of age, with open interdental spaces

* 4 molar and 4 incisor interdental test sites per subject, identified as "an Inter-Dens could be passed easily from the facial to the lingual aspects, a minimum of 1 cm from the tip"

* 3 consecutive study periods of 1 week each (cross-over design):
    - Manual toothbrush + waxed dental floss
    - Manual toothbrush + balsawood triangular stick (Inter-Dens firm)
    - Manual toothbrush + single tufted brush (Interspace)

* At baseline, subjects received prophylaxis (plaque score = 0) and instructed to supplement their normal toothbrushing with twice daily interdental cleaning using assigned regimen for 1st week

* Recordings, prophylaxis and instruction with another regimen after 1 week; repeated 1 week later to allow all subjects to use all 3 regimens

* Interdental plaque scores of test teeth using disclosing dye and Wolffe index (presence/absence in 4 subdivisions of the interdental surfaces below the contact point; bucco-coronal, bucco-apical, linguo-coronal, linguo-apical; maximum score = 4 when all 4 'quadrants' of the interdental surface show plaque)

* Comparisons of mean plaque scores at the end of each 1-week period for subgroups of interdental surfaces

Results:

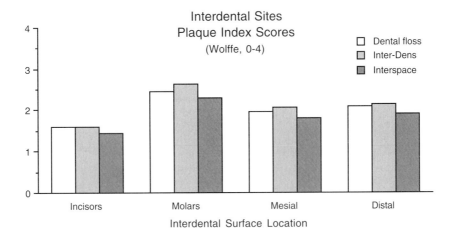

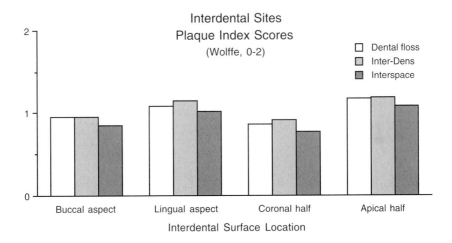

Comments:

- Although average interdental cleaning was incomplete, interdental plaque scores for incisors were lower than for molars. Buccal aspects of interdental surfaces showed slightly lower scores than lingual aspects, and coronal half of interdental surfaces slightly lower than apical half. (Note that the maximum score is 2 for buccal/lingual and coronal/apical aspects, since only half of the interdental surface and 2 'quadrants' are included.)

- For all interdental surface locations, similar plaque scores were observed following use of all 3 cleaning methods.

- The author remarked: "There was a considerable range of individual plaque scores. Those who cleaned well with one agent, cleaned well with the other two. Examination of individual plaque scores demonstrated that the same areas were missed each week."

- A 4th study group - use of toothbrush alone - would have been desirable.

- Bergenholtz et al. (1974) compared interdental cleaning of open embrasures using dental floss, round toothpicks, rectangular toothpicks and triangular woodsticks. It was observed that round and rectangular toothpicks were effective on buccal but not on lingual aspects of interdental surfaces, whereas triangular woodsticks and dental floss were effective on both buccal and lingual aspects.

- Bergenholtz et al. (1980) compared interdental plaque removal in open embrasures following use of triangular woodsticks made of balsa, birch and lime, and did not find any systematic differences between the 3 materials.

KIGER ET AL. (1991) evaluated plaque removal efficacy of dental floss and an interdental brush in open interdental embrasures.

Subjects and procedures:

* 30 adult patients with open interdental spaces, under maintenance following previous periodontal treatment

* Previous use of interdental cleaning aids not ascertained

* 2-4 interdental test sites per subject, identified as "embrasures sufficiently open to allow easy passage of an interdental brush"

* 3 consecutive study periods of 1 month each (cross-over design):
    - Manual toothbrush alone
    - Manual toothbrush + unwaxed dental floss
    - Manual toothbrush + interdental brush (Oral-B)

* Following baseline recordings, subjects received prophylaxis (plaque score = 0) and instruction in toothbrushing and in interdental cleaning with assigned regimen (if any) for 1st month; interdental aid, toothbrush and dentifrice provided

* Recordings, prophylaxis and instruction with another regimen after 1 month; repeated 1 month later to allow all subjects to use all 3 regimens

* Plaque scores of test teeth after use of disclosing gel:
    - Buccal/lingual aspects of the teeth with Turesky/Quigley-Hein index (scores 0-5)
    - Interdental plaque scores of test teeth using disclosing dye and Wolffe index (presence/absence in 4 subdivisions of the interdental surfaces below the contact point; bucco-coronal, bucco-apical, linguo-coronal, linguo-apical; maximum score = 4 when all 4 'quadrants' of the interdental surface show plaque)

* Comparison of mean plaque scores at the end of each 1-month period for buccal/lingual and interdental sites

Results:

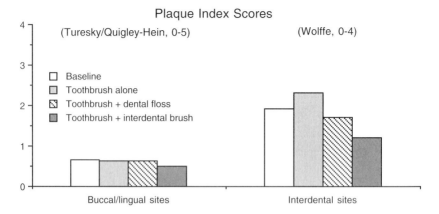

Comments:

- Buccal/lingual plaque scores were low prior to prophylaxis at baseline and were also low at the end of each experimental 1-month period.

- Mean interdental plaque scores following use of toothbrush alone were somewhat higher than those prior to prophylaxis at baseline, suggesting that at least some patients might have practiced interdental cleaning prior to the study.

- Although still incomplete, interdental plaque control was more effective following use of the interdental brush as compared to use of floss. The average Wolffe plaque index score around 1 for the interdental brush means that overall, the patients showed stained plaque in one of the 4 'quadrants' of the interdental surfaces.

- The authors also evaluated soft tissue trauma and stated that it "was noted in only isolated areas and was unrelated to the use of floss or interdental brushes".

- This study is supported by results of 3 other studies on plaque control of interdental surfaces in open interdental spaces. Gjermo & Flötra (1970) found an interdental brush more effective than dental floss and triangular woodsticks. Nayak & Wade (1977) found an interdental brush more effective than an interdental rubber cone stimulator. Bergenholtz & Olsson (1984) found all of 3 tested interdental brushes more effective than waxed dental floss.

Interdental cleaning

Concluding remarks

Use of dental floss can reduce plaque levels on proximal surfaces and contribute to improved gingival health. Little or no difference in efficacy has been found between various floss types. Use of floss aids does not appear to provide increased effectiveness. This includes an electrically powered interdental cleaner, which seems to be equally good, but no more effective than finger flossing.

In open embrasures, wide enough for use of interdental brushes, these brushes seem to be somewhat more efficient than other interdental aids.

Triangular woodsticks are also effective in reducing interdental gingivitis. There seem to be no studies on the possibility of a cosmetic disadvantage in visible maxillary areas following introduction of woodsticks as compared to floss, i.e. if woodstick use will result in increased papillary recession and thereby causing larger open embrasures than the use of floss.

Available studies demonstrate that, on average, proximal/interdental plaque control is still suboptimal in the participating subjects. This may be related to motivation and compliance aspects as well as deficiencies of the available tools. Irrespective of the reason for this less than ideal proximal/interdental plaque control, the results call for new and more effective interdental cleaning methods.

Studies on interdental cleaning should carefully separate included subjects and sites with respect to presence of intact periodontal tissues (no reduction of papillary height) versus presence of open interdental embrasures (reduced papillary height).

In many studies, dental plaque has been scored following use of a disclosing dye and with indices that will record minimum amounts of plaque (e.g. Turesky/Quigley-Hein). It should be kept in mind that it may not be possible to reach a score of 0 with this system, if the teeth have not been professionally cleaned at study baseline, since firmly adhering deposits with limited bacterial content may absorb some stain. However, studies with professional tooth cleaning at baseline have also shown suboptimal interdental plaque control (e.g. Wolffe, 1976 and Kiger et al. 1991, pages 58-62).

Although only some studies on interdental cleaning have reported that individuals with impaired dexterity have been excluded from participation, it may be assumed that the subjects generally have had no dexterity disadvantage?

Unfortunately, studies on interdental cleaning are short-term. Long-term results comparing various aids may be different than short-term results due to variation in patient acceptance of the various tools.

Interdental cleaning

References

Abelson, D.C., Barton, J.E., Maietti, G.M. & Cowherd, M.G. (1981) Evaluation of interproximal cleaning by two types of dental floss. Clinical Preventive Dentistry 3 (4), 19-21.

Barton, J. & Abelson, D. (1987) The clinical efficacy of wooden interdental cleaners in gingivitis reduction. Clinical Preventive Dentistry 9 (6), 17-20.

Barton, R. & Diamond, B. (1980) Evaluation and patient acceptance of a mechanical dental flossing device compared to hand-held floss. Clinical Preventive Dentistry 2 (3), 10-12.

Bergenholtz, A. & Brithon, J. (1980) Plaque removal by dental floss or toothpicks. An intraindividual comparative study. Journal of Clinical Periodontology 7, 516-524.

Bergenholtz, A. & Olsson, A. (1984) Efficacy of plaque-removal using interdental brushes and waxed dental floss. Scandinavian Journal of Dental Research 92, 198-203.

Bergenholtz, A., Bjorne, A. & Vikström, B. (1974) The plaque-removing ability of some common interdental aids. An intraindividual study. Journal of Clinical Periodontology 1, 160-165.

Bergenholtz, A., Bjorne, A., Glantz, P-O. & Vikström, B. (1980) Plaque removal by various triangular toothpicks. Journal of Clinical Periodontology 7, 121-128.

Carter-Hanson, C., Gadbury-Amyot, C. & Killoy, W. (1996) Comparison of the plaque removal efficacy of a new flossing aid (Ouik Floss) to finger flossing. Journal of Clinical Periodontology 23, 873-878.

Ciancio, S.G., Shibley, O. & Farber, G.A. (1992) Clinical evaluation of the effect of two types of dental floss on plaque and gingival health. Clinical Preventive Dentistry 14 (3), 14-18.

Cronin, M. & Dembling, W (1996) An investigation of the efficacy and safety of a new electric interdental plaque remover for the reduction of interproximal plaque and gingivitis. Journal of Clinical Dentistry 7, 74-77.

Cronin, M., Dembling, W. & Warren, P. (1997) The safety and efficacy of gingival massage with an electric interdental cleaning device. Journal of Clinical Dentistry 8, 130-133.

Gjermo, P. & Flötra, L. (1970) The effect of different methods of interdental cleaning. Journal of Periodontal Research 5, 230-236.

Gordon, J.M., Frascella, J.A. & Reardon, R.C. (1996) A clinical study of the safety and efficacy of a novel electric interdental cleaning device. Journal of Clinical Dentistry 7, 70-73.

Graves, R.C., Disney, J.A. & Stamm, J.W. (1989) Comparative effectiveness of flossing and brushing in reducing interproximal bleeding. Journal of Periodontology 60, 243-247.

Kiger, R.D., Nylund, K. & Feller, R.P. (1991) A comparison of proximal plaque removal using floss and interdental brushes. Journal of Clinical Periodontology 18, 681-684.

Kleber, C.J. & Putt, M.S. (1988) Evaluation of a floss-holding device compared to hand-held floss for interproximal plaque, gingivitis and patient acceptance. Clinical Preventive Dentistry 10 (4), 6-14.

Lamberts, D.M., Wunderlich, R.C. & Caffesse, R.G. (1982) The effect of waxed and unwaxed dental floss on gingival health. Part I. Plaque removal and gingival response. Journal of Periodontology 53, 393-396.

Lobene, R.R., Soparkar, P.M. & Newman, M.B. (1982) Use of dental floss. Effect on plaque and gingivitis. Clinical Preventive Dentistry 4 (1), 5-8.

Nayak, R.P. & Wade, A.B. (1977) The relative effectiveness of plaque removal by the Proxabrush and rubber cone stimulator. Journal of Clinical Periodontology 4, 128-133.

Ong, G. (1990) The effectiveness of 3 types of dental floss for interdental plaque removal. Journal of Clinical Periodontology 17, 463-466.

Pucher, J., Jayaprakash, P., Aftyka, T., Sigman, L. & Van Swol, R. (1995) Clinical evaluation of a new flossing device. Quintessence International 26, 273-278.

Spindel, L. & Person, P. (1987) Floss design and effectiveness of interproximal plaque removal. Clinical Preventive Dentistry 9 (3), 3-6.

Spolsky V.W., Perry, D.A., Meng, Z. & Kissel, P. (1993) Evaluating the efficacy of a new flossing aid. Journal of Clinical Periodontology 20, 490-497.

Stevens, A.W. (1980) A comparison of the effectiveness of variable diameter vs. unwaxed dental floss. Journal of Periodontology 51, 666-667.

Wolffe, G.N. (1976) An evaluation of proximal surface cleansing agents. Journal of Clinical Periodontology 3, 148-156.

Wong, C.H. & Wade, A.B. (1985) A comparative study of effectiveness in plaque removal by SuperFloss and waxed dental floss. Journal of Clinical Periodontology 12, 788-795.

SECTION 4

Electric toothbrushes

Electric toothbrushes were introduced half a century ago. Most powered brushes on the market over the years have had vibratory, reciprocating or arcuate movements of the brush heads, simulating the small scrubbing movements often recommended for manual brushing. Studies on the efficacy of these electric brushes have not provided any clear evidence to indicate that these brushes are superior to manual brushing.

More recently, powered toothbrushes using different brush head motions have been introduced and renewed the interest. The majority of available studies on these powered brushes in groups of patients have used observation periods limited to 3-6 weeks. Interpretation of such short-term results is confounded by the possibility of a 'novelty effect' of the electric brushes. As referred to before, subjects using a newly invented product may be more attentive and thorough using this device during an initial period than the familiar use of a conventional product, thereby favoring the results for the new device. Therefore, short-term studies have not been included in this section. Longer term studies are available on the relative efficacy of 4 brushes compared to manual brushing (Braun Oral-B Plak Control, Interplak, Rota-dent and Sonicare). For each of these brushes, a study in adults is reviewed.

A single-use study in dental students comparing one of the brushes (Braun Oral-B Plak Control) to manual toothbrushing has been included to provide an example of the relative efficacy under 'optimal conditions'.

STUDIES PRESENTED IN THIS SECTION

Authors	Page	Subjects	Brushes evaluated	Observation interval
van der Weijden et al. (1993)	69	Dental students	Braun Oral-B Manual	Single-use
Ainamo et al. (1997)	71	Adults with gingivitis	Braun Oral-B Manual	12 months
Tritten & Armitage (1996)	75	Adults with gingivitis	Sonicare Manual	3 months
Wilson et al. (1993)	79	Adults with gingivitis	Interplak Manual	12 months
Boyd et al. (1989)	84	Periodontal maintenance patients	Rota-dent Manual + interdental aids	12 months

VAN DER WEIJDEN (1993) compared Braun Oral-B Plak Control to manual toothbrushing in a single-use study.

Subjects and procedures:
* 20 dental students without previous experience of powered toothbrushes

* 3 consecutive phases of experimentation:
    Phase 1: professional brushing
    - Students asked to refrain from toothbrushing for 24 hours prior to test

    - Prebrushing plaque scores, followed by brushing by a professional, followed by postbrushing plaque scores

    - Diagonal quadrants brushed with Braun Oral-B Plak Control and Butler GUM 311 (split-mouth design)

    - Brushing time = 30 seconds/quadrant; no toothpaste; method of manual brushing not reported

    - *Phase 2: brushing by the subjects*
      - Students given written instructions on use of Braun Oral-B Plak Control and on Bass method of manual toothbrushing, and asked to practice the 2 methods on alternate days during 3 weeks

      - Students asked to abstain from toothbrushing for 24 hours prior to test

      - Prebrushing plaque scores, followed by supervised brushing by the subjects themselves, followed by postbrushing plaque scores

      - Diagonal quadrants brushed with Braun Oral-B Plak Control and Butler GUM 311 (split-mouth design)

      - Brushing time = 30 seconds/quadrant; standard toothpaste

    - *Phase 3: brushing by the subjects following additional instruction and prophylaxis*
      - Students given personal 'hands-on' instructions on use of Braun Oral-B Plak Control and on Bass method of manual toothbrushing, and asked to continue practicing the 2 methods on alternate days during 3 weeks

      - Students given dental prophylaxis (plaque scores = 0) and asked to abstain from toothbrushing for 48 hours prior to test

      - Plaque scores and supervised brushing as for Phase 2

* Plaque scores at 6 locations of each tooth using Silness-Löe index (scores 0-3)

Results:

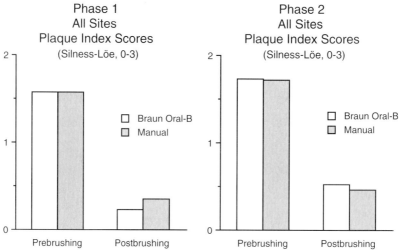

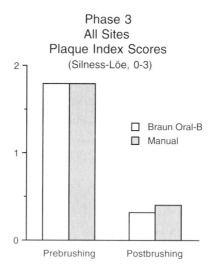

Comments:

- Plaque scores were markedly reduced from prebrushing to postbrushing for all 3 phases of experimentation. Only small differences in reductions between the electric and manual brushes were noted. (The differences in Phase 1 and Phase 3 in favor of the electric brush reached statistical significance, whilst the difference in favor of the manual brush in Phase 2 did not.)

- The reductions of plaque scores in this single-use study in dental students are considerably greater than the prebrushing to postbrushing reductions observed following manual or powered toothbrushing in patient groups (compare Yankell et al. 1996, page 37; Tritten & Armitage 1996, page 77; Wilson et al. 1993, page 81).

AINAMO ET AL. (1997) compared the use of Braun Oral-B Plak Control to manual toothbrushing over 12 months.

Subjects and procedures:
* 111 office-workers, 20-63 years of age, with full mouth bleeding on probing scores ≥30% (details on any attachment loss/interdental papillary heights not provided)

* Study groups matched for age, sex, plaque scores, bleeding scores and use/no use of interdental hygiene aids (parallel design):
    - Braun Oral-B Plak Control electric toothbrush (N=55)
    - Manual toothbrush, Jordan soft (N=56)

* After baseline recordings, subjects received prophylaxis (plaque scores = 0) and instructions in brushing techniques (Braun Oral-B Plak Control/modified Bass); no additional instruction during the observation interval

* Instructions to brush mornings and evenings for 2 minutes using a provided standard toothpaste; continued use of interdental aids allowed

* Recordings from all maxillary right and mandibular left teeth ('half-mouth')

* Presence/absence of visible dental plaque at the gingival margin recorded for 4 sites per tooth (mesio-buccal, mid-buccal, disto-buccal and lingual; % sites with plaque)

* Presence/absence of bleeding on probing recorded at 6 sites per tooth (% sites with bleeding)

* 12 months of observation

* Analyses:
    1) Mean plaque and bleeding scores for all examined surfaces
    2) Mean plaque and bleeding scores for subgroups of surfaces:
        - Maxillary anterior, buccal and lingual aspects
        - Maxillary posterior, buccal and lingual aspects
        - Mandibular anterior, buccal and lingual aspects
        - Mandibular posterior, buccal and lingual aspects

Results:

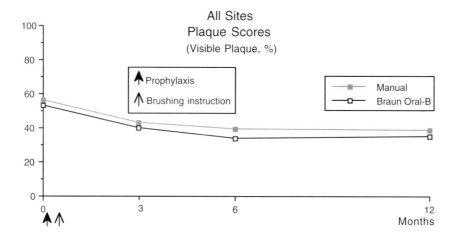

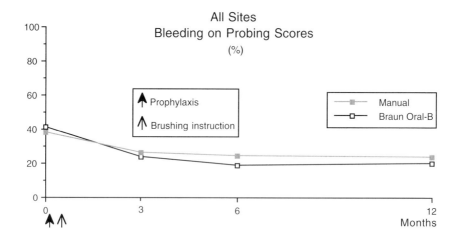

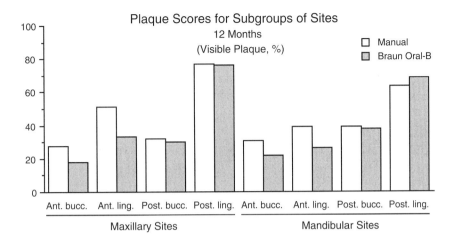

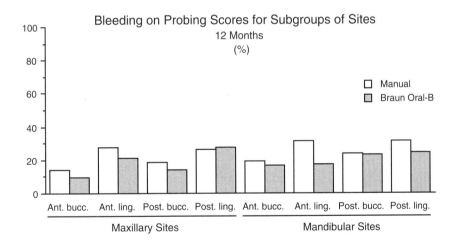

Comments:

- Both groups showed reduced overall plaque and bleeding scores after 3 months. Slight additional changes were observed thereafter. The changes from baseline to 3 months may have been caused by the initial prophylaxis, at least in part.

- Separation of the 12-month plaque and bleeding scores on different surface types revealed lower scores for the electric brush than the manual brush for anterior buccal and lingual surfaces. Plaque scores remained particularly high for posterior lingual surfaces.

- It should be pointed out that plaque scores for buccal aspects included both mid-surface and proximal surfaces. Separate analyses for proximal surfaces, both from the buccal and lingual aspects, would have been of interest, as would separate analyses for subjects using/not using interdental aids.

- This study, thus, found some benefits to Braun Oral-B Plak Control over manual brushing. The largest difference was observed for the lingual aspects of the anterior teeth, where 71% of sites were free of bleeding for the manual brush at 12 months as compared to 81% for the electric brush. The results are supported by observations of van der Weijden et al. (1994) who compared Braun Oral-B Plak Control to manual brushing over 8 months in university students. They observed an advantage to Braun Oral-B Plak Control, primarily for mid-buccal and proxo-buccal surfaces. No advantage was noted for mid-lingual and proxo-lingual surfaces.

- In another study, Braun Oral-B Plak Control was compared to manual brushing in adult gingivitis patients during 3 months (Barnes et al. 1993). Plaque scores were presented for all surfaces and separately for proximal surfaces and showed no change for either the electric or manual group. Gingivitis scores for these 2 surface groups showed no change for the manual brush, but a minimal improvement for the electric brush for both surface groups.

- Thus, the above studies in gingivitis patients indicate that overall, Braun Oral-B Plak Control may be slightly superior to manual brushes for plaque and gingivitis control. However, the results are not clear as to the particular surfaces that might benefit from the use of this brush.

- In the study by van der Weijden et al. (1994) (referred to above) patients were inspected for gingival abrasion at 4 examinations over the 8 months of study. A total of 12 incidents of abrasion were found for the manual group and 7 for the Braun Oral-B Plak Control group.

TRITTEN & ARMITAGE (1996) compared Sonicare to manual toothbrushing.

Subjects and procedures:

* 56 patients, 22-59 years of age, with gingivitis but with no probing depth ≥6 mm (details on any attachment loss/interdental papillary heights not provided)

* Study groups (parallel design):
  - Sonicare electric toothbrush (N=29)
  - Manual toothbrush, Butler #311 (N=27)

* After baseline recordings, subjects instructed in brushing techniques during 10 minutes (Sonicare/modified Bass), followed by monitored brushing during 2 minutes, followed by renewed plaque recording

* No baseline prophylaxis

* Instructions to brush mornings and evenings for 2 minutes using a provided standard toothpaste, and to refrain from use of other oral hygiene aids during the first month of study

* Instructions not to brush for 12-14 hours before each follow-up visit to allow assessment of overnight plaque

* Pre- and postbrushing plaque recordings repeated at examinations after 1 and 3 months

* Plaque scores at 6 sites of each tooth using disclosing dye and Turesky/Quigley-Hein index (scores 0-5)

* Presence/absence of bleeding on probing recorded at 6 sites for each of 6 representative teeth in the dentition ('Ramfjord teeth'[†]) (% sites with bleeding)

* 3 months of observation

* Analyses:
  - Mean plaque scores for various groups of surfaces
  - Mean bleeding scores for examined teeth

[†] See Appendix 2: Glossary of Experimental Designs (pages 279-291).

Results:

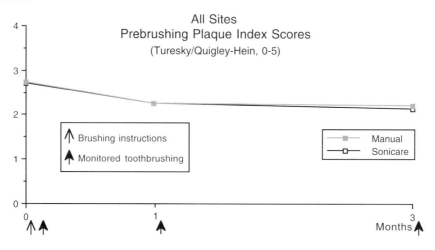

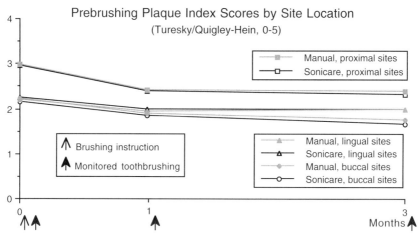

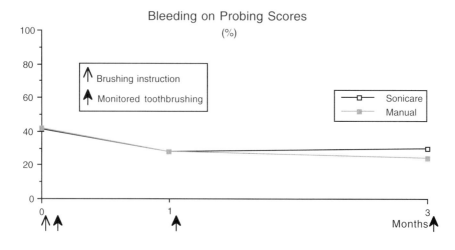

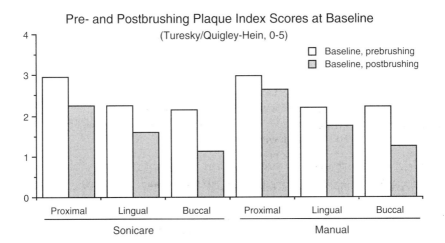

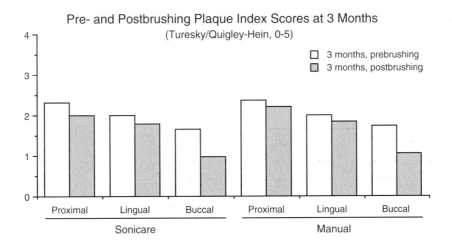

Comments:

- Compared to baseline, both brushing groups showed reduced prebrushing plaque scores after 1 month for all evaluated site types. Additional reduction between 1 to 3 months was only observed for buccal sites. Little difference was observed between electric and manual brushing over the 3-month observation interval.

- Bleeding scores also improved from baseline to 1 month with no further change and without any difference between study groups.

- The brushings at the examination visits reduced the overnight plaque levels, particularly for buccal sites. Pre- to postbrushing reductions were greater at baseline than at 1 and 3 months (only baseline and 3 months shown here), presumably due to the larger amounts of plaque present at baseline. At baseline, a slightly improved pre- to postbrushing reduction for proximal and lingual sites was observed for the electric compared to the manual brush. At 1 and 3 months, pre- to postbrushing reductions were modest for proximal and lingual sites.

- The permission to use other oral hygiene aids starting at 1 month had little impact as evidenced by the similarity of scores at 1 and 3 months.

- Although this study showed a trend in favor of Sonicare for baseline plaque removal at proximal and lingual sites, the difference was marginal and without a concomitant difference over the 3 months of study for any of 3 clinical parameters of gingival inflammation (only results of bleeding scores presented here).

- The subjects continued to show fairly high plaque scores during the 3 months in spite of their participation in the study. 71% (Sonicare) and 79% (manual) of all postbrushing scores were index scores ≥ 2 (i.e. a minimum of a thin continuous band of plaque at the cervical margin; see Appendix 1: Commonly Used Plaque and Gingival Indices; Turesky/Quigley-Hein plaque index, page 271).

- Patients were also inspected for gingival abrasion at each examination. A total of 6 incidents of abrasion were observed for the manual group and 1 for the Sonicare group.

WILSON ET AL. (1993) compared Interplak to manual toothbrushing.

Subjects and procedures:

* 29 adults with plaque scores ≥50% and gingivitis, but with no probing depth ≥7 mm (details on any attachment loss/interdental papillary heights not provided)

* Study groups (parallel design):
    - Interplak electric toothbrush (N=13)
    - Manual toothbrush, Butler #311 (N=16)

* Prophylaxis completed before baseline (time point not given)

* After baseline recordings, subjects instructed in brushing techniques (Interplak/modified Bass), followed by unsupervised brushing during 3 minutes, followed by renewed plaque recording

* Instructions to use a provided dentifrice and to refrain from use of other oral hygiene aids

* Instructions to brush 1 hour before each follow-up visit

* Pre- and postbrushing plaque recordings and brushing instruction repeated after 1 week and 1, 2, 6, 9 and 12 months

* Plaque scores at 6 sites of each tooth using disclosing dye and Turesky/Quigley-Hein index (scores 0-5)

* Bleeding on sulcular probing (gentle horizontal scraping) recorded at 6 sites of each tooth using Barnett/Mühlemann index (quickness of bleeding, scores 0-3)

* 12 months of observation

* Analyses of mean plaque and bleeding scores for various groups of sites

Results:

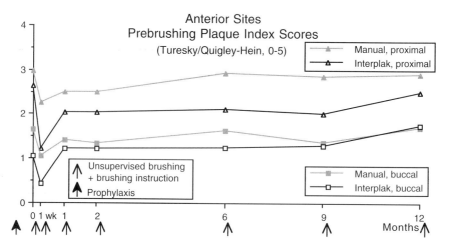

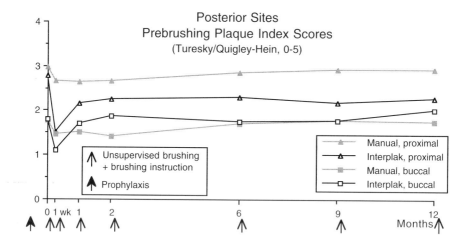

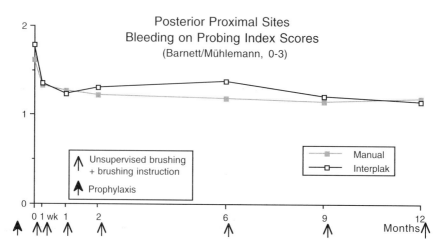

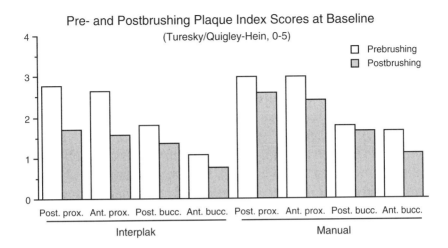

Pre- and Postbrushing Plaque Index Scores at Baseline
(Turesky/Quigley-Hein, 0-5)

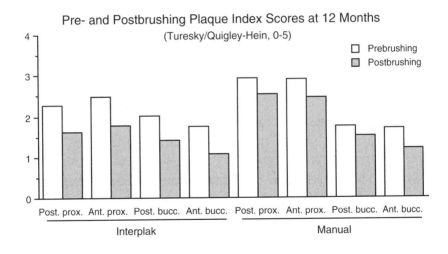

Pre- and Postbrushing Plaque Index Scores at 12 Months
(Turesky/Quigley-Hein, 0-5)

Comments:

- Transient improvements of prebrushing plaque scores were observed after 1 week. Anterior and posterior proximal sites seemed to show less plaque following use of electric than manual brush throughout the 12 months of observation, although the groups were not properly matched at baseline. Little or no difference between groups were noted for buccal sites. The authors did not present any data for lingual sites, but remarked that they did not differ from buccal sites.

- Bleeding scores for all subgroups of sites improved similarly for both brushing groups during the 1st month of study (only posterior proximal sites shown here). These improvements may have been influenced by the prophylaxis provided prior to baseline. Little change was noted between 1 and 12 months. Thus, although proximal plaque scores were lower for the electric than the manual brush throughout the study, there was no corresponding difference for proximal bleeding scores.

- The brushings at the examinations reduced the plaque levels, more so for electric than manual brush (only baseline and 12-month scores shown here).

- This study included a limited number of subjects. They continued to show comparatively high plaque scores during the 12 months of study in spite of the repeated instructions and examinations.

- Gingival abrasion was recorded at each examination using an abrasion index (data not shown here). The authors concluded that "little or no abrasion was observed in either group".

- Yukna & Shaklee (1993) compared Interplak without supplementary interdental aids to manual tooth cleaning including use of interdental aids in patients under maintenance following previous periodontal treatment. Proximal plaque scores (presence/absence) over 6 months of observation decreased from 59% to 41% for the manual group and from 61% to 30% for the Interplak group. This suggests that the patients could maintain a certain degree of proximal plaque control by using the Interplak brush without the use of interdental aids.

- In a study by Quirynen et al. (1993), Interplak and a manual brush were compared in a small number of patients treated for moderate periodontitis. Dentifrice and other oral hygiene aids were not used with either brush. After 6 months and use of Interplak, 65-70% of proximal sites harbored plaque, as compared to 80-90% following use of manual brush. These numbers also indicate a modest effect of Interplak at proximal locations.

- In both of these studies on periodontitis patients by Yukna & Shaklee (1993) and Quirynen et al. (1994), details on extent of open embrasures were not provided. Thus, it is not clear to what degree the proximal scores of these studies represent interdental sites, i.e. sites underneath the contact point of open embrasures.

BOYD ET AL. (1989) compared Rota-dent to manual tooth cleaning.

Subjects and procedures:

* 35 patients, 24-69 years of age, under maintenance following previous peri-odontal treatment, including periodontal surgery (details on extent of open interdental embrasures not provided)

* Study groups matched for age, sex and gingival inflammation (parallel design):
  - Rota-dent electric toothbrush, 3 brush heads (cup-shaped + pointed + long-pointed); discontinued use of interdental aids (N=18)
  - Manual toothbrush, Oral-B; continued use of interdental aids - details not given (N=17)

* 1 week after baseline recordings, subjects received maintenance treatment including supra- and subgingival debridement and instructions in brushing techniques (Rota-dent/modified Bass)

* Instructions to brush twice daily using a provided standard dentifrice

* Renewed instructions after 1, 3, 6 and 9 months; repeated maintenance treatment after 6 months

* Recordings from proximal sites of 6 representative teeth in the dentition ('Ramfjord teeth'); 3 mesio-buccal + 3 disto-buccal sites

* Presence/absence of visible dental plaque at the gingival margin (% sites with plaque); presence/absence of bleeding on probing (% sites with bleeding)

* 12 months of observation

* Analyses of mean plaque and bleeding scores

Results:

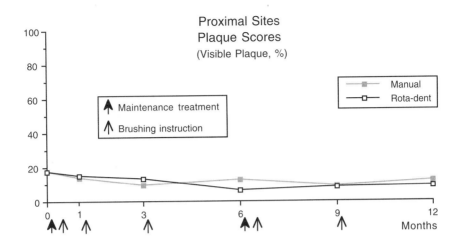

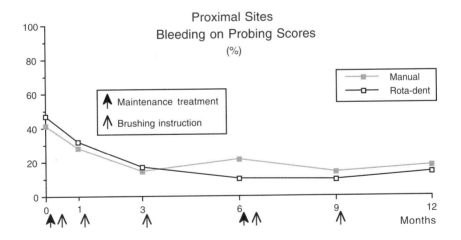

Comments:

- Plaque scores for the selected mesio-buccal and disto-buccal sites were comparatively low at baseline and showed only a slight and similar improvement for both groups.

- Bleeding scores for the selected sites improved similarly for the 2 groups during the initial 3 months. The improvements, at least in part, may have been caused by the maintenance treatment at baseline.

- The results indicate that periodontal maintenance patients, most likely having some open interdental embrasures, can maintain a similar degree of proximal plaque control by using the Rota-dent brush heads instead of manual toothbrush + interdental aids. Recordings for linguo-proximal sites would have been of interest.

- The authors reported that "no gingival abrasions were noted on any subjects from either study group at any of the clinical examinations".

- The results of this study are supported by the findings of Glavind & Zeuner (1986). In 2 groups of patients, treated nonsurgically for periodontal disease, Rota-dent was compared to conventional brush + interdental aids. Full mouth plaque and bleeding scores were presented and demonstrated corresponding improvements for both groups after 3 months (plaque scores reduced from 58-59% to 19-21%; bleeding scores reduced from 51-53% to 22-23%).

- The extent of presence of open embrasures in the subjects of Boyd et al. (1989) and Glavind & Zeuner (1986) was not reported. Thus, and again, it is not clear to what degree the proximal scores represent interdental sites, i.e. sites below the contact point of open embrasures. The actual use of interdental aids in the manual cleaning groups was neither reported. These shortcomings need to be considered for the interpretation of the findings.

Electric toothbrushes

Concluding remarks

Although available studies do not allow a complete evaluation, use of Braun Oral-B Plak Control, Interplak and Sonicare electric toothbrushes may facilitate tooth cleaning compared to manual brushes. However, the degree of advantage for each of these electric brushes over manual brushes seems limited. It is questionable if the daily use of the electric brushes in patient groups over study periods of 3-12 months has resulted in any improvement of gingival conditions compared to manual brushing that would be of clinical importance.

Braun Oral-B Plak Control and Sonicare brushes have been compared to each other in separate studies. Grossman et al. (1995), in a 2-month study in gingivitis patients, found no differences between the devices. Robinson et al. (1997), treating patients with mild to moderate periodontitis, found similar reductions of plaque scores, but slightly greater reductions of bleeding scores over 6 months for the Sonicare than for the Braun Oral-B Plak Control.

Use of Rota-dent and its 3 brush heads may provide a similar degree of cleaning as manual brush + interdental aids. However, details on effects on interdental sites have not been reported.

The participants of the studies reviewed have most likely been limited to subjects with normal dexterity, although this has not been stated in the papers.

In a survey among recall patients of a periodontal specialty clinic, it was found that 36 months after purchase, 62% of patients were still using the electric toothbrush on a daily basis (Stålnacke et al. 1995). Apart from this report, little is known about the continued use of electric toothbrush following their recommendation.

The incidence of gingival abrasion may not be higher following use of electric than manual brushes. Development of gingival recession and cervical root surface abrasion does not seem to have been investigated following electric toothbrushing, and may take several years of exposure for adequate evaluation.

As mentioned before, many studies on toothbrushing effectiveness would have been easier to interpret, if:

- subjects and sites to be included had been carefully selected with respect to intact versus reduced interdental papillary height;

- data on % plaque-free and % gingivitis-free proximal/interdental sites had been presented.

Electric toothbrushes

References

Ainamo, J., Xie, Q., Ainamo, A. & Kallio, P. (1997) Assessment of the effect of an oscillating/rotating electric toothbrush on oral health. A 12-month longitudinal study. Journal of Clinical Periodontology 24, 28-33.

Barnes, C.M., Weatherford, T.W. & Menaker, L. (1993) A comparison of the Braun Oral-B plaque remover (D5) electric and a manual toothbrush in affecting gingivitis. Journal of Clinical Dentistry 4, 48-51.

Boyd, R.L., Murray, P. & Robertson, P.B. (1989) Effect on periodontal status of rotary electric toothbrushes vs. manual toothbrushes during periodontal maintenance. I. Clinical results. Journal of Periodontology 60, 390-395.

Glavind, L. & Zeuner, E. (1986) The effectiveness of a rotary electric toothbrush on oral cleanliness in adults. Journal of Clinical Periodontology 13, 135-138.

Grossman, E., Dembling, W. & Proskin, H.M. (1995) A comparative clinical investigation of the safety and efficacy of an oscillating/rotary electric toothbrush and a sonic toothbrush. Journal of Clinical Dentistry 6, 108-112.

Quirynen, M., Vervliet, E., Teerlinck, J., Darius, P. & van Steenberghe, D. (1994) Medium- and long-term effectiveness of a counterrotational electric toothbrush on plaque removal, gingival bleeding, and probing pocket depth. International Journal of Periodontics and Restorative Dentistry 14, 365-377.

Robinson, P.J., Maddalozzo, D. & Breslin, S. (1997) A six-month clinical comparison of the efficacy of the Sonicare and the Braun Oral-B electric toothbrushes on improving periodontal health in adult periodontitis patients. Journal of Clinical Dentistry 8, 4-9.

Stålnacke, K., Söderfeldt, B. & Sjödin. B. (1995) Compliance in use of electric toothbrushes. Acta Odontologica Scandinavia 53, 17-19.

Tritten, C.B. & Armitage G.C. (1996) Comparison of a sonic and a manual toothbrush for efficacy in supragingival plaque removal and reduction of gingivitis. Journal of Clinical Periodontology 23, 641-648.

van der Weijden, G.A., Danser, M.M., Nijboer, A., Timmerman, M.F. & van der Welden, Ü (1993) The plaque-removing efficacy of an oscillating/rotating toothbrush. A short-term study. Journal of Clinical Periodontology 20, 273-278.

van der Weijden, G.A., Timmerman, M.F., Reijerse, E., Danser, M.M., Mantel, M.S., Nijboer, A. & van der Velden, Ü. (1994) The long-term effect of an oscillating/rotating electric toothbrush on gingivitis. An 8-month clinical study. Journal of Clinical Periodontology 21, 139-145.

Wilson, S., Levine, D., Dequincey, G. & Killoy, W.J. (1993) Effects of two toothbrushes on plaque, gingivitis, gingival abrasion, and recession: a 1-year longitudinal study. Compendium on Continued Education in Dentistry, suppl. 16, s569-s579.

Yukna, R.A. & Shaklee, R.L. (1993) Interproximal vs midradicular effects of a counter-rotational powered brush during supportive periodontal therapy. Compendium on Continued Education in Dentistry, suppl. 16, s580-s586.

SECTION 5

Frequency of tooth cleaning

How often should people clean their teeth? Ideally, this section should provide scientific evidence to justify recommendations - general or individualized - on how often toothbrushing and interdental cleaning ought to be performed in order to prevent or reduce dental caries and periodontal disease.

Theoretically, prospective experimental studies could be designed in individuals with various susceptibility to caries and periodontal disease. Within a particular category of patients, experimental groups could be allocated to different frequencies of tooth cleaning, e.g. 1 x daily, 2 x daily and 3 x daily. Development of caries and periodontal disease could then be evaluated and compared. Such trials, however, would be coupled with extreme difficulty. For example, they need to have observation periods of several years in order to provide useful data on disease progression. A significant compliance problem would be involved - how can it be assured that the participating subjects will adhere to the assigned frequency of cleaning over periods of several years? In addition, ethical reasons will not permit the use of experimental groups allocated to frequencies of cleaning which potentially may involve disease progression, based upon current prevailing opinions.

Since gingivitis may develop within a few weeks and is reversible, prospective studies on cleaning frequency and gingivitis have been carried out. The minimum frequency of tooth cleaning needed to prevent development of gingivitis has been investigated in 2 similar experimental studies. One of these studies is reviewed.

STUDY PRESENTED IN THIS SECTION

Authors	Page	Subjects	Frequency of tooth cleaning	Observation interval
Lang et al. (1973)	93	Dental students	2 x daily Every 2nd day Every 3rd day Every 4th day	6 weeks

LANG ET AL. (1973) studied the frequency of tooth cleaning needed to prevent the development of gingivitis.

Subjects and procedures:
* 32 dental students with healthy gingiva

* 4 study groups with various tooth cleaning frequency (parallel design, 'experimental gingivitis' model):
    - 2 x daily (N=8)
    - Every 2nd day (N=8)
    - Every 3rd day (N=8)
    - Every 4th day (N=8)

* Supervised cleanings using toothbrush, dental floss and interdental wood-sticks; complete plaque removal verified by a professional using disclosing dye (for 2 x daily group, supervision during one of the daily cleanings only)

* Gingivitis scores at 4 locations of each tooth using Löe-Silness index (scores 0-3)

* 6 weeks of observation

* Analyses of mean gingivitis scores

Results:

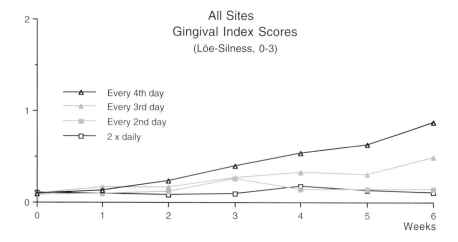

Comments:

- Brushing + interdental cleaning twice daily and also once every 2nd day prevented development of gingivitis, whilst cleaning every 3rd and every 4th day did not.

- In a similar study in dental students/young dental faculty, tooth cleanings practiced once daily and once every 3rd day were compared. Development of gingivitis was prevented by cleaning once daily, but not by cleaning once every 3rd day (Kelner et al. 1974).

- The minimum frequency of tooth cleaning needed to reverse experimentally induced gingivitis has also been investigated in dental students. Oral hygiene procedures were abandoned in sections of the mouth during 21 days in order to induce gingivitis, followed by their reinstitution. Cleaning once daily and also once every 2nd day was sufficient to reverse the gingivitis, whilst cleaning every 3rd day was not (Bosman & Powell 1977).

Frequency of tooth cleaning

Concluding remarks

Tooth cleanings once daily and also once every 2nd day have been found to prevent the development of gingivitis in dental students. Although interesting as
such, these studies may have limited clinical relevance. Most patients are not
able to achieve total plaque removal at each cleaning, like these dentally motivated subjects.

Another approach has been attempted to evaluate tooth cleaning frequency. Self-
reported frequency of tooth cleaning has been related to exposure to caries and
periodontal disease in cross-sectional studies of various populations. Results for
the relationship to caries have been equivocal (see review by Bellini et al. 1981,
Murtomaa et al. 1984). A more recent study was carried out in a random sample
of 35-year-olds from Oslo, Norway (when fluoridated dentifrices constituted the
main share of the market). Both frequency of toothbrushing and oral hygiene
status were included among factors related to the number of decayed surfaces.
Whilst the degree of oral cleanliness showed a weak but statistically significant
relationship to number of carious surfaces, the frequency of toothbrushing
showed no association (Bjertness 1991).

The results of studies on the relationship between tooth cleaning frequency and
periodontal disease have also been variable (e.g. Dale 1969, Horton et al. 1969,
Hansen & Johansen 1977, Murtomaa et al. 1984, Hansen et al. 1990, Lang et al.
1995). In a study of adults living in the area of Detroit, USA, Lang et al. (1995)
found that plaque scores and observed brushing thoroughness were better linked
to periodontal conditions than brushing frequency. Regular use of dental floss
and observed flossing ability also related to periodontal conditions.

Thus, cross-sectional studies associating tooth cleaning frequency to caries and
periodontal disease may mainly indicate that the quality of cleaning relates more
to disease than the frequency of cleaning.

In spite of the lack of scientific background, a general recommendation to clean
the teeth twice daily, morning and evening, is common. This direction is
conceivably based on reasons of practicability and feeling of oral freshness,
rather than reasons of disease control based upon research data.

Frequency of tooth cleaning

References

Bellini, H.T., Arneberg, P. & von der Fehr, F.R. (1981) Oral hygiene and caries. A review. Acta Odontologica Scandinavia 39, 257-265.

Bjertness, E. (1991) The importance of oral hygiene on variation in dental caries in adults. Acta Odontologica Scandinavia 49, 97-102.

Bosman, C.W. & Powell, R.N. (1977) The reversal of localized experimental gingivitis. Journal of Clinical Periodontology 4, 161-172.

Dale, J.W. (1969) Toothbrushing frequency and its relationship to dental caries and periodontal disease. Australian Dental Journal, April, 120-123.

Hansen, B.F. & Johansen, J.R. (1977) Periodontal treatment needs of 35-year-old citizens in Oslo. Journal of Clinical Periodontology 4, 263-271.

Hansen, B.F., Bjertness, E. & Gjermo, P. (1990) Changes in periodontal disease indicators in 35-year-old Oslo citizens from 1973 to 1984. Journal of Clinical Periodontology 17, 249-254.

Horton, J.E., Zimmermann, E.R. & Collings, C.K. (1969) The effect of toothbrushing frequency on periodontal disease measurements. Journal of Periodontology 40, 14-16.

Lang, N.P., Cumming, B.R. & Löe, H. (1973) Toothbrushing frequency as it relates to plaque development and gingival health. Journal of Periodontology 44, 396-405.

Lang, W.P., Ronis, D.L. & Farghaly, M.M. (1995) Preventive behaviours as correlates of periodontal health status. Journal of Public Health Dentistry 55, 10-17.

Kelner, R.M., Wohl, B.R., Deasy, M.J. & Formicola, A.J. (1974) Gingival inflammation as related to frequency of plaque removal. Journal of Periodontology 45, 303-307.

Murtomaa, H., Turtola, L. & Rytömaa, I. (1984) Differentiating positively and negatively health oriented Finnish university students by discriminant analyses. Community Dentistry and Oral Epidemiology 12, 243-248.

SECTION 6

Subgingival cleaning

The Bass method of toothbrushing seems to be widely recommended. One of the reasons for this recommendation may be its potential to accomplish some degree of subgingival reach and cleaning. Although cleaning below the gingival margin may not be necessary to maintain already healthy gingival conditions, subgingival cleaning would seem to be advantageous once subgingival plaque has formed and a gingivitis/periodontitis process has developed.

A few studies have been performed on condemned, periodontally diseased teeth scheduled for extraction. Prior to extraction, the teeth have been brushed and a groove has been placed along the gingival margin. The distance between the apical portion of the groove and the coronal border of the remaining subgingival plaque has been measured following extraction and used as an indication of the depth of subgingival cleaning.

Another indication of subgingival cleaning effectiveness may be gleaned from studies evaluating the effect of personal plaque control procedures on periodontal pockets of different depths. What depths of pockets can be resolved by personal plaque control alone, without supplementary professional subgingival debridement?

STUDIES PRESENTED IN THIS SECTION

Authors	Page	Procedure	Treatment	Evaluation
Youngblood et al. (1985)	99	Brushing prior to extraction of peri-odontally diseased teeth	Manual brushing Electric brushing Unbrushed control	Depth of sub-gingival plaque removal
Rapley & Killoy (1994)	101	Brushing prior to extraction of peri-odontally diseased teeth	Manual brushing Electric brushing Unbrushed control	Depth of sub-gingival plaque removal
Cercek et al. (1983)	103	Treatment of peri-odontal pockets of various depths	Personal plaque con-trol alone versus professional subgin-gival debridement	Bleeding on probing and probing depth changes

YOUNGBLOOD ET AL. (1985) studied the depth of subgingival plaque removal following manual and electric brushing.

Subjects and procedures:

* 55 periodontally diseased teeth scheduled for extraction, having at least one proximal surface in contact with an adjacent tooth

* Minimum probing depth not required; mean depth around 3.5 mm

* Teeth to be extracted brushed by a professional on buccal and lingual aspects using assigned brush, 10 seconds each

* Treatment groups:
    - Manual brushing using Bass method (toothbrush type not reported) (25 teeth)
    - Electric brushing using Interplak toothbrush as recommended by manufacturer (25 teeth)
    - Unbrushed control (5 teeth)

* Following brushing, grooves placed along buccal and lingual gingival margins

* Extraction, followed by plaque staining and measurement of distance between apical portion of groove and coronal portion of remaining subgingival plaque at 6 locations: mid-buccal, mesio-buccal and disto-buccal line angles, mid-lingual, and mesio-lingual and disto-lingual line angles

Results:

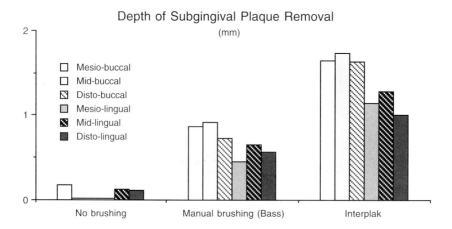

Comments:

- Although the number of unbrushed control teeth was very limited, subgingival plaque was found close to the gingival margin groove.

- Results following manual brushing showed a range of mean depths of subgingival plaque removal from 0.5 to 0.9 mm. On average, plaque removal seemed deeper for buccal than for lingual aspects.

- Results following brushing with Interplak showed a range of mean depths of subgingival plaque removal from 1.0 to 1.7 mm. Again, deeper removal was observed for buccal than for lingual aspects.

- It should be reiterated that the 'proximal' measurements were obtained at the line angles.

- The authors remarked that some of the electrically brushed specimens did not show any remaining subgingival plaque coronal to the level of connective tissue attachment. In these cases, depth of cleaning was measured to the connective tissue level and may have included the plaque-free zone (usually present coronal to the attachment and 0.5-1.5 mm wide). This "would have served to exaggerate the depth to which plaque was removed in those cases." For these specimens, the authors could have opted to reduce the measurements with the average width of the plaque-free zone as observed from the other specimens. This would probably have provided a better representation of the depth of subgingival plaque removal.

RAPLEY & KILLOY (1994) also studied the depth of subgingival plaque removal following manual and electric brushing.

Subjects and procedures:

* 90 periodontally diseased teeth scheduled for extraction, showing buccal, mesial and lingual probing depths ≥5 mm and bleeding on probing

* Details on presence of adjacent teeth not given

* Teeth to be extracted brushed by a professional on buccal and lingual aspects, 10 seconds each

* Treatment groups:
    - Manual brushing using Bass method and Reach soft toothbrush (30 teeth)
    - Electric brushing using Braun Oral-B Plak Control toothbrush as recommended by manufacturer (30 teeth)
    - Unbrushed control (30 teeth)

* Following brushing, grooves placed along buccal and lingual gingival margins

* Extraction, followed by plaque staining and measurement of distance between apical portion of groove and coronal portion of remaining subgingival plaque at 6 locations: mid-buccal, mesio-buccal and disto-buccal line angles, mid-lingual, and mesio-lingual and disto-lingual line angles

Results:

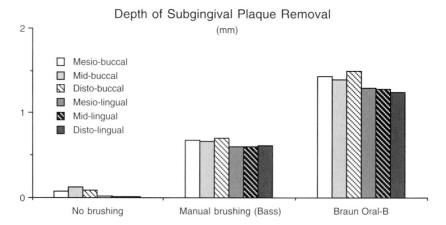

Depth of Subgingival Plaque Removal
(mm)

Legend:
- ☐ Mesio-buccal
- ☐ Mid-buccal
- ☒ Disto-buccal
- ▨ Mesio-lingual
- ▧ Mid-lingual
- ■ Disto-lingual

Categories: No brushing, Manual brushing (Bass), Braun Oral-B

Comments:

- The findings from unbrushed control teeth verified the presence of subgingival plaque close to the gingival margin.

- Results following manual brushing showed a range of depth of subgingival plaque removal from 0.6 to 0.7 mm.

- Results following brushing with Braun Oral-B Plak Control showed a range of depth of subgingival plaque removal from 1.3 to 1.5 mm.

- The results parallel those of Youngblood et al. (1985) (pages 99-100) and indicate a certain depth of subgingival reach and plaque removal following manual brushing using Bass method, but a more noticeable removal following use of Interplak and Braun Oral-B Plak Control electric brushes.

- The findings of these 2 studies, using professional brushing and mid-surface and line angle measurements, are contrasted by the observations of Taylor et al. (1995). They studied proximal subgingival locations next to contacting adjacent teeth following brushings performed by patients after brief instructions. Subgingival cleaning could not be observed following use of either Interplak or Braun Oral-B Plak Control electric brushes. Following manual brushing, average depth of subgingival cleaning amounted to 0.5 mm, although quite some variation was observed among the few specimens studied.

CERCEK ET AL. (1983) studied the relative effects of personal plaque control alone and plaque control combined with professional supra- and subgingival debridement.

Subjects and procedures:

* 7 patients with moderate to advanced periodontitis

* Only incisors, cuspids and bicuspids included for study

* Periodontal pockets ≥5 mm deep with subgingival calculus and bleeding upon probing at 2 or more surfaces of each experimental tooth

* 3 consecutive phases of treatment:
    - Phase 1 (0-5 months): Plaque control using toothbrush and dental floss
    - Phase 2 (5-8 months): Perio-Aid added for subgingival use during home care (a round, pointed toothpick mounted on a handle for sulcular use by the patients)
    - Phase 3 (8-17 months): A single episode of professional supra- and sub-gingival instrumentation given at 8 months

* Recordings at 6 sites per tooth:
    - plaque scores (presence/absence, %)
    - bleeding scores (presence/absence, %)
    - probing depths (mm)

* Analysis of results for sites with initial depth:
    ≤3.5 mm
    4-5.5 mm
    ≥6 mm

Results:

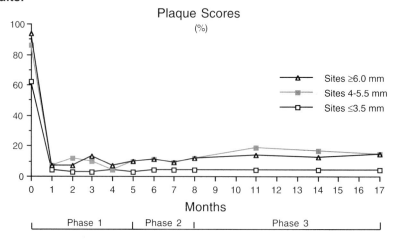

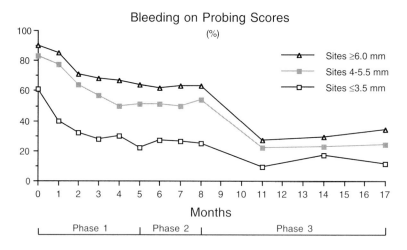

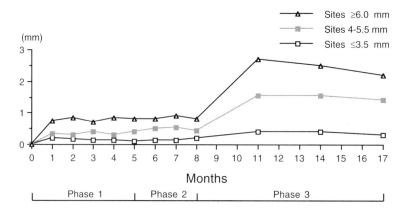

Comments:

- The average level of personal plaque control was high in this study on a small number of patients. Low plaque scores were obtained for all sites of the investigated nonmolar teeth, irrespective of initial probing depth.

- During the first couple of months of Phase 1 - use of toothbrush and dental floss - bleeding scores improved for all 3 categories of initial probing depths. The relative reduction was greatest for the shallow sites.

- Some reduction of probing depth occurred during the first month of Phase 1. This was more noticeable for deeper pockets.

- The introduction of Perio-Aid in Phase 2 did not seem to affect the recorded parameters. The Perio-Aid may not have allowed access to the subgingival areas. Lack of compliance to the recommended use may also have been involved.

- Professional instrumentation resulted in additional improvement, primarily for sites initially 4-5.5 mm and ≥6 mm. In other words, personal plaque control alone for these sites provided only a limited portion of the total improvement. The results of this study are in accordance with several other studies, and may indirectly suggest that the extent of subgingival reach of personal plaque control procedures is limited (e.g. Listgarten et al. 1978, Lindhe et al. 1983, Wennström et al. 1987 and Heijl et al. 1991).

Subgingival cleaning

Concluding remarks

Subgingival cleaning following toothbrushing to a depth of 1.0 - 1.5 mm may be possible under favorable circumstances - electric brushes operated by professionals at accessible buccal and lingual sites. Subgingival plaque removal following brushing by patients, however, may be more limited and requires additional study.

Subgingival cleaning by various interdental cleaning aids does not seem to have been systematically studied in humans, although case series of extracted teeth have demonstrated the potentials for subgingival plaque removal following use of interdental brushes and dental floss (Waerhaug 1975, 1978, 1981).

Noticeable clinical improvements can be observed in sites with shallow pocket depth following personal plaque control procedures alone. This may not, however, be related to any significant subgingival reach and cleaning. Removal of plaque initially located subgingivally may be a gradual process due to reduced gingival edema and gradual supragingival exposure of the plaque.

Subgingival cleaning

References

Cercek, J.F., Kiger, R.D., Garrett, S. & Egelberg, J. (1983) Relative effects of plaque control and instrumentation on the clinical parameters of periodontal disease. Journal of Clinical Periodontology 10, 46-56.

Heijl, L., Dahlén, G., Wenander, Y. & Goodson, J.M. (1991) A 4-quadrant comparative study of periodontal treatment using tetracycline-containing drug delivery fibers and scaling. Journal of Clinical Periodontology 18, 111-116.

Lindhe, J., Linjenberg, B., Adielsson, B. & Börjesson, I. (1983) Use of metronidazole as a probe in the study of human periodontal disease. Journal of Clinical Periodontology 10, 100-112.

Listgarten, M.A., Lindhe, J. & Helldén, L. (1978) Effect of tetracycline and/or scaling on human periodontal disease. Journal of Clinical Periodontology 5, 246-271.

Rapley, J.W. & Killoy, W.J. (1994) Subgingival and interproximal plaque removal using a counter-rotational electric toothbrush and a manual toothbrush. Quintessence International 25, 39-42.

Taylor, J.Y., Wood, C.L., Garnick, J.J. & Thompson, W.O. (1995) Removal of interproximal subgingival plaque by hand and automatic toothbrushes. Journal of Periodontology 66, 191-196.

Waerhaug, J. (1975) The interdental brush and its place in operative and crown and bridge dentistry. Journal of Oral Rehabilitation 3, 107-113.

Waerhaug, J. (1978) Healing of the dento-epithelial junction following subgingival plaque control. II. As observed on extracted teeth. Journal of Periodontology 49, 119-134.

Waerhaug, J. (1981) Healing of the dento-epithelial junction following the use of dental floss. Journal of Clinical Periodontology 8, 144-150.

Wennström, J.L., Heijl, L., Dahlén, G. & Gröndahl, K. (1987) Periodic subgingival antimicrobial irrigation of periodontal pockets. I. Clinical observations. Journal of Clinical Periodontology 14, 541-550.

Youngblood, J.J., Killoy, W.J., Love, J.W. & Drisko, C. (1985) Effectiveness of a new home plaque-removal instrument in removing subgingival and interproximal plaque: a preliminary in vivo report. Compendium of Continuing Education, suppl. 6, s128-141.

Toothbrushing trauma

Gingival abrasion/ulceration, gingival recession and cervical abrasion of the root surface may develop as unwanted side effects of toothbrushing.

Data on gingival recession from 2 different Scandinavian groups of individuals with regular dental attendance and comparatively good standard of oral hygiene suggest that (Löe et al. 1992, Serino et al. 1994):

- Around 5% of buccal surfaces of 20-year-olds and 25% of buccal surfaces of 40-year-olds display ≥1 mm of gingival recession;

- Gingival recession is less frequent for lingual surfaces, about 8% in 40-year-olds;

  In 20-30 year-olds gingival recession is most frequent for buccal surfaces of maxillary premolars and 1st molars and mandibular premolars;

- In 30-40 year-olds recession has become more common also for buccal surfaces of other tooth groups.

Although some of this recession may be related to periodontitis, it is likely that the majority of the recession defects in the younger individuals is associated with trauma from toothbrushing.

Cervical abrasion may occur once the root surface has been exposed by gingival recession. The distribution of cervical abrasion in the mouth, therefore, seems to mirror that of gingival recession (Sangnes & Gjermo 1976, review by Sangnes 1976).

To provide examples, this section reviews a few studies investigating some factors related to development of gingival abrasion, gingival recession and cervical root surface abrasion. In addition, a few other studies are quoted and listed on the following page to provide a more complete description of factors found associated with these lesions.

STUDIES PRESENTED IN THIS SECTION

Authors	Page	Subjects	Injury	Injury-related factors
Niemi et al. (1984)	111	Dental hygiene students	Gingival abrasion	Toothbrush stiffness Dentifrice abrasiveness
Breitenmoser et al. (1979)*	113	18-28 year-olds	Gingival abrasion	End-cut of toothbrush filaments
Khocht et al. (1993)	114	18-56 year-olds	Gingival recession	Toothbrush stiffness Brushing frequency
Mierau & Spindler (1984)*	115	25-year-olds	Gingival recession	Brushing time Brushing force
Paloheimo et al. (1987)*	115	17-20 year-olds	Gingival recession	Rate of toothbrush wear
Källestål & Uhlin (1992)*	115	18-year-olds	Buccal attachment loss	Buccal tooth displacement Thickness of buccal alveolar tissue
Bergström & Lavstedt (1979)	116	Sample of city population	Cervical abrasion	Brushing method Brushing frequency Toothbrush stiffness Dentifrice abrasiveness
Radentz et al. (1976)*	118	Dental technician trainees	Cervical abrasion	Toothbrush stiffness Quantity of dentifrice Sequence of brushing

* Study not reviewed, findings quoted.

NIEMI ET AL. (1984) examined the frequency of gingival lesions following brushing with toothbrushes of various stiffness and toothpastes with different abrasiveness.

Subjects and procedures:
* 24 dental hygiene students, 22-34 years of age, with healthy gingiva

* 3 consecutive, split-mouth experiments, each separated by 1 week (total of 6 study groups):
    - Soft toothbrush (Sensodyne, filament diameter 0.15 mm); no dentifrice
    - Soft toothbrush + moderately abrasive dentifrice (Pepsodent Fluor)
    - Soft toothbrush + highly abrasive dental powder (Smokers)
    - Hard toothbrush (Te-Pe, filament diameter 0.23 mm); no dentifrice
    - Hard toothbrush + moderately abrasive dentifrice
    - Hard toothbrush + highly abrasive dental powder

* Subjects asked to refrain from oral hygiene procedures 2 days before each test

* Subjects' teeth brushed during 1 minute per half mouth by one and the same dental hygienist using modified Bass method

* Gingival abrasions/lacerations/ulcerations recorded at 4 aspects of each tooth

* Plaque scores of buccal and lingual aspects of all teeth using disclosing dye and Bay & Ainamo index (degree of plaque extension over the tooth surface; scores 0-3)

* Comparisons of:
    - postbrushing frequencies of gingival lesions
    - postbrushing plaque scores

Results:

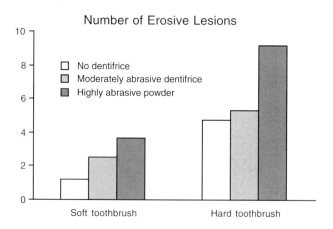

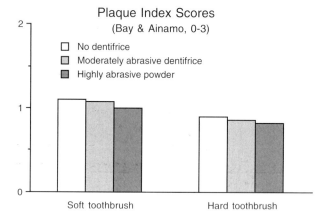

Comments:

- The mean number of gingival lesions was higher following use of the hard brush than the soft brush. In addition, for each of the brushes, the number of lesions was related to the abrasiveness of the dentifrice/powder.

- The postbrushing plaque scores indicated a trend that increased stiffness of the toothbrush filaments and increasing abrasiveness of the dentifrice resulted in lower amounts of residual plaque (score 1 = small flecks or short strands of stained plaque along the gingival margin). Regrettably, prebrushing scores were not reported, which would have facilitated the interpretation.

- Also, data on brushing force and the amounts of dentifrice/powder used would have been desirable.

- The soft brush used for the study, having 0.15 mm filament diameter, represent the softest brushes on the market. Still, some abrasive lesions were observed. This may, at least partly, be related to the sensitivity of the scoring method used (although details were not presented, the authors had previously verified the reliability of their clinical scoring method through comparisons with scanning electron micrographs of impressions/replicas; Sandholm et al. 1982).

- The possibility of differences in rounding of the filament ends of the brushes used was not commented upon. This may have had some relevance for the gingival abrasions, since new brushes were used. Alexander et al. (1977) using hamster cheek pouches mounted on a brushing apparatus, found less abrasion after use of end-rounded filaments than use of filaments without end-rounding. (In addition, using this model, less abrasion was observed after lower compared to higher brushing force and after softer compared to harder brushes.) Breitenmoser et al. (1979) evaluating gingival abrasion in students brushing in a standardized fashion also observed less abrasion following use of rounded as compared to nonrounded filaments.

KHOCHT ET AL. (1993) related gingival recession to brushing frequency and hard toothbrush use.

Subjects and procedures:

* 182 volunteers, 18-56 years of age, at 2 clinical dental research facilities

* Interview for information on:
    - Age
    - Brushing frequency
    - Filament stiffness (soft, medium, hard)

* Clinical examination of buccal and lingual aspects of all teeth for gingival recession (presence/absence)

* Analysis of the relationship between hard toothbrush use, brushing frequency and % surfaces with gingival recession

Results:

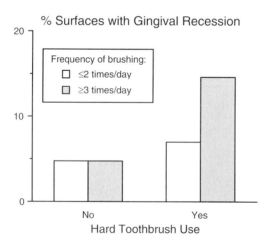

Comments:

- Individuals using hard toothbrushes showed a higher frequency of surfaces with gingival recession than individuals reported to use medium or soft brushes. In addition, among those using hard brushes gingival recession was related to toothbrushing frequency.

- As expected, gingival recession was found to increase with age (data not shown here). Hard toothbrush use was not related to age, and therefore did not confound the findings.

- Findings from some additional studies on gingival recession should be added in this context:

    i) Miereau & Spindler (1984), studying subjects around 25 years of age, found that individuals with gingival recession used longer brushing time and greater brushing force than individuals without recession.

    ii) Paloheimo et al. (1987) found that gingival recession in 17-20 year-olds was related to rate of toothbrush wear. Thus, 70% of the adolescents reporting a service life of their toothbrushes <2 months exhibited recession as compared to 22% of those reporting a service life >6 months.

    iii) Källestål & Uhlin (1992) found that buccal attachment loss in 18-year-olds was associated with buccal tooth displacement and thin buccal alveolar tissues (hard + soft). This confirms previous observations by Gorman (1967) that tooth malalignment is associated with gingival recession.

BERGSTRÖM & LAVSTEDT (1979) related the incidence of cervical abrasions to toothbrushing characteristics in an adult population.

Subjects and procedures:
* 818 individuals representing the adult population of Stockholm, Sweden

* Cervical, root surface abrasions classified as:
    - Superficial lesion: "clearly visible and explorable abrasion"
    - Deep lesion: "clearly identifiable wedge-shaped defect"

* Number of individuals using various toothbrushing habits determined by observation/interview

* Toothbrushing method:
    - Horizontal strokes (N=124)
    - Vertical strokes (N=333)
    - Combination horizontal/vertical (N=246)
    - Roll technique (N=115)

* Toothbrushing frequency:
    - Less than once a day (N=29)
    - Once a day (N=124)
    - Twice a day (N=510)
    - More than twice a day (N=155)

* Toothbrush stiffness:
    - Soft (N=73)
    - Medium (N=394)
    - Hard (N=351)

* Dentifrice abrasivity:
    - Low (N=96)
    - Medium (N=374)
    - High (N=348)

* Analyses of % subjects with ≥1 superficial and/or deep lesions and with ≥1 deep lesions for subgroups of age, sex and toothbrushing characteristics

Results:

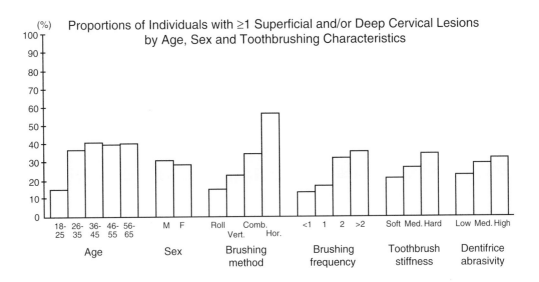

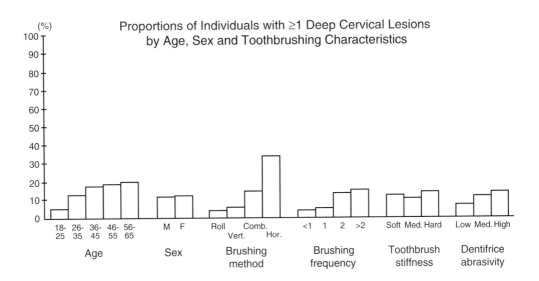

Comments:

- Toothbrushing method showed the strongest association with cervical abrasion. Individuals using the roll method showed the lowest, and individuals using horizontal strokes the highest occurrence of abrasion.

- Brushing frequency also showed a noticeable relationship to abrasion. Less association was found for toothbrush stiffness and dentifrice abrasivity. These latter characteristics, however, may not have been stable over the years.

- Radentz et al. (1976) compared toothbrushing habits for 2 groups of dental technician trainees - with and without presence of cervical abrasion. They found that individuals with abrasion used larger quantities of dentifrice and hard brushes more often than individuals without abrasion. The authors also found that 58% of all abrasions were present in those 3 areas of the dentition observed to be brushed first as compared to 42% of abrasions for the remaining 13 investigated areas of the dentition.

- A few prospective studies on cervical abrasion have been conducted, using observation periods ranging from 1 to 4.5 years (Volpe et al. 1975, Saxton & Cowell 1981, Nordbø & Skogedal 1982).The degree of cervical abrasion in the examined individuals/teeth has generally been found to increase over the observation intervals. Attempts have been made to relate this increase to the abrasiveness of the dentifrices used, as determined from the *in vitro* abrasive values of these dentifrices. Within the range of abrasive values investigated, however, little or no relationship between *in vitro* and *in vivo* abrasiveness has been found. It appears that cervical abrasion is not easily attributed to individual, single factors and may be the result of a combination of contributory factors.

Toothbrushing trauma

Concluding remarks

Several oral hygiene related factors have been found to be associated with presence of gingival recession on buccal aspects of teeth: hard toothbrush use, brushing frequency, brushing time, brushing force and rate of toothbrush wear. These factors may all be part of vigorous or overzealous toothbrushing inducing trauma to the gingival tissues.

The pathogenesis of traumatically induced gingival recession has not been clarified. The recession process needs to include 2 events: apical recession of the gingival margin and loss of connective tissue attachment from the root surface. Hypothetically, repeated abrasions/ulcers of the gingival margin and the subsequent healing processes may cause a shrinkage of the marginal gingival tissue ('scar formation') and initiate a recession. The cause of attachment loss seems more difficult to speculate upon, but might possibly be related to a genetically inherent need for a certain height of the unattached gingival cuff (a concept which is supported by studies on healing events following gingivectomy). A reduction of the height of the unattached portion of the gingiva below a certain level might initiate a compensatory remodelling. Compensation for shrinkage of the marginal gingiva following repeated injury and upholding of a gingival cuff may only be possible through detachment of connective tissue fibers from the root surface.

Cervical abrasion may develop from superficial lesions into wedge shape defects. Frequent brushings, horizontal brushing strokes, use of hard toothbrush and a highly abrasive dentifrice seem to be a combination of factors with abrasive potentials. The relative importance of these factors has not been clarified. Nevertheless, both soft and hard tissue lesions seem related to ardent toothbrushing.

Case presentations have illustrated both interdental soft tissue lesions and proximal root surface abrasion associated with overzealous use of interdental cleaning aids. However, there seems to be no systematic study on interdental lesions in adults.

Toothbrushing trauma

References

Alexander, J.F., Saffir, A.J. & Gold, W. (1977) The measurement of the effect of toothbrushes on soft tissue abrasion. Journal of Dental Research, 56, 722-727.

Bergström, J. & Lavstedt, S. (1979) An epidemiologic approach to toothbrushing and dental abrasion. Community Dentistry and Oral Epidemiology 7, 57-64.

Breitenmoser, J., Mörmann, W. & Mühlemann, H.R. (1979) Damaging effects of toothbrush bristle end form on gingiva. Journal of Periodontology 50, 212-216.

Gorman, W.J. (1967) Prevalence and etiology of gingival recession. Journal of Periodontology 38, 316-322.

Khocht, A., Simon, G., Person, P. & Denepitiya, J.L. (1993) Gingival recession in relation to history of hard toothbrush use. Journal of Periodontology 64, 900-905.

Källestål, C. & Uhlin, S. (1992) Buccal attachment loss in Swedish adolescents. Journal of Clinical Periodontology 19, 485-491.

Löe, H., Ånerud, Å. & Boysen, H. (1992) The natural history of periodontal disease in man: Prevalence, severity, and extent of gingival recession. Journal of Periodontology 63, 489-495.

Mierau, H-D. & Spindler, T. (1984) Beitrag zur Ätiologie der Gingivarezesssionen. Deutsche Zahnärztliche Zeitschrift 39, 634-639.

Niemi, M-L., Sandholm, L. & Ainamo, J. (1984) Frequency of gingival lesions after standardized brushing as related to stiffness of toothbrush and abrasiveness of dentifrice. Journal of Clinical Periodontology 11, 254-261.

Nordbø, H. & Skogedal, O. (1982) The rate of cervical abrasion in dental students. Acta Odontologica Scandinavica 40, 45-47.

Paloheimo, L., Ainamo, J., Niemi, M-L. & Viikinkoski, M. (1987) Prevalence of and factors related to gingival recession in Finnish 15- to 20-year old subjects. Community Dental Health 4, 425-436.

Radentz, W.H., Barnes, G.P. & Cutright, D.E. (1976) A survey of factors possibly associated with cervical abrasion of tooth surfaces. Journal of Periodontology 47, 148-154.

Sandholm, L., Niemi, M-L. & Ainamo, J. (1982) Identification of soft tissue brushing lesions. A clinical and scanning microscopic study. Journal of Clinical Periodontology 9, 397-401.

Sangnes, G. (1976) Traumatization of teeth and gingiva related to habitual tooth cleaning procedures. Journal of Clinical Periodontology 3, 94-103.

Sangnes, G. & Gjermo, P. (1976) Prevalence of oral soft and hard tissue lesions related to mechanical toothcleansing procedures. Community Dentistry and Oral Epidemiology 4, 77-83.

Saxton, C.A. & Cowell, C.R. (1981) Clinical investigation of the effects of dentifrices on dentin wear at the cementoenamel junction. Journal of the American Dental Association 102, 38-43.

Serino, G., Wennström, J., Lindhe, J. & Eneroth, L. (1994) The prevalence and distribution of gingival recession in subjects with a high standard of oral hygiene. Journal of Clinical Periodontology 21, 57-63.

Volpe, A.R., Mooney, R., Zumbrunnen, C., Stahl, D. & Goldman, H.M. (1975) A long term clinical study evaluating the effect of two dentifrices on oral tissues. Journal of Periodontology 46, 113-118.

SECTION 8

Tongue brushing

The dorsum of the tongue harbors a great number of microorganisms. These bacteria may serve as a source of bacterial dissemination to other parts of the oral cavity, e.g. the tooth surfaces. Therefore, tongue brushing has been advocated as an adjunct to toothbrushing, since this might reduce formation of dental plaque by means of reducing a potential reservoir of microorganisms contributing to plaque formation. This section includes reviews of 4 studies identified within this topic, 3 of them published during the 1970's and 1 during the 1980's.

The bacterial accumulations on the dorsum of the tongue may also be a source of mouth odor, especially after awakening in the morning. During sleep, reduced muscular activity and reduced salivary flow may favor microbial growth and retention on the tongue in particular. Tongue brushing has been recommended to reduce early morning mouth odor. This section includes 1 study on this problem.

STUDIES PRESENTED IN THIS SECTION

Authors	Page	Outcome variable	Cleaning supple-ment/methods	Experimental conditions
Jacobson et al. (1973)	125	Plaque formation	Tongue + palate brushing Control	2 weeks of habitual toothbrushing 2 days without tooth cleaning
Gross et al. (1975)	127	Plaque formation	Tongue brushing Control	6 weeks of habitual toothbrushing
Badersten et al. (1975)	129	Plaque formation	Tongue brushing Control	4 days without tooth cleaning 7 days with restric-ted toothbrushing
Rowley et al. (1987)	131	Plaque formation	Tongue brushing Tongue scraping Control	2 weeks of habitual toothbrushing
Tonzetich & Ng (1976)	133	Oral odorous substances	Toothbrushing Tongue brushing Tooth + tongue brushing Control	Morning mouth odor

JACOBSON ET AL. (1973) studied the effect of brushing the tongue + palate on plaque formation.

Subjects and procedures:
* 30 adults, 21-32 years of age, with normal periodontium

* 2 study cycles (cross-over design), each including 2 weeks of habitual tooth brushing followed by 2 days of no tooth cleaning:
    - Tongue + palate brushing, 2 x daily during 1 minute
    - Control: no tongue + palate cleaning

* Following baseline examination, all subjects received prophylaxis (plaque score = 0), toothbrush and toothpaste, asked to brush twice daily with a dentifrice in their usual manner, and to refrain from use of mouthwash

* Plaque scores from all teeth after 2 weeks using disclosing dye and Löe-Silness index (scores 0-3)

* Repeated prophylaxis followed by 2 days without tooth cleaning + repeated plaque scores

* Analyses of mean plaque scores

Results:

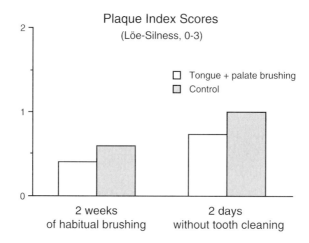

Comments:

- Lower mean plaque scores were observed following use of supplementary tongue + palate brushing, both after 2 weeks of habitual brushing and 2 days without tooth cleaning.

- At the end of the 2-week habitual brushing periods, the authors also determined the amounts of oral debris collected in 1 liter of expectorate following use of a water-pressure irrigation device directed at the tongue and palate. They found that tongue + palate brushing reduced the amount of debris by 35% (data not shown here).

GROSS ET AL. (1975) evaluated the effect of tongue brushing as a supplement to toothbrushing on plaque formation in 2 identical studies.

Subjects and procedures:
* Enlisted military men, 17-31 years of age

* Study 1 groups, matched for baseline plaque scores (parallel design):
    - Tongue brushing, 5 strokes from posterior to anterior (N=25)
    - Control: no tongue brushing (N=21)

* Study 2 groups, matched for baseline plaque scores (parallel design):
    - Tongue brushing, 5 strokes from posterior to anterior (N=57)
    - Control: no tongue brushing (N=51)

* Following baseline examination, all subjects received prophylaxis (plaque score = 0), a soft toothbrush, and asked to continue their normal oral hygiene procedures

* Plaque scores from buccal and lingual aspects of all teeth using disclosing dye and Quigley-Hein index (scores 0-5)

* Degree of coating on the dorsum of the tongue evaluated with index (scores 0-3; none, slight, moderate, heavy)

* 6 weeks of observation

* Analyses of mean plaque and tongue coating scores

Results:

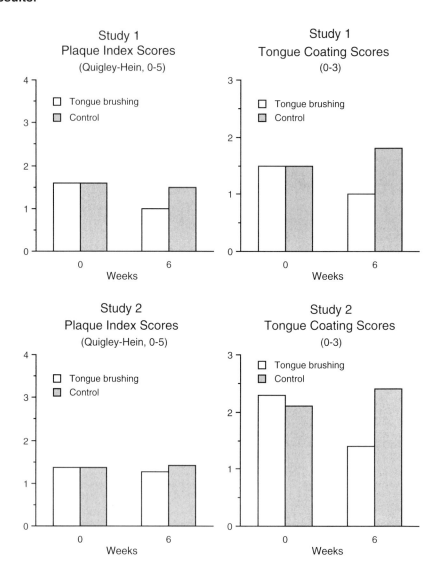

Comments:

- After 6 weeks of habitual toothbrushing, mean plaque scores corresponded to baseline scores prior to prophylaxis. Reduced plaque levels were observed following tongue brushing in Study 1, but not in Study 2.

- The degree of tongue coating was reduced following tongue brushing in both studies. The overall higher coating scores in Study 2 compared to Study 1 may possibly relate to examiner drift.

BADERSTEN ET AL. (1975) studied the effect of tongue brushing on plaque formation during a 4-day period of no tooth cleaning and during a 7-day period of restricted toothbrushing.

Subjects and procedures:
* 2 different groups of 8 dental hygiene students each, 24-44 years of age

* Study 1 (4 days of no tooth cleaning):
    Experimental groups (cross-over design):
    - Tongue brushing, 3 x daily, 5 strokes per tongue quadrant, no dentifrice (mid-day brushing supervised)
    - Control: no tongue brushing

    At baseline, all subjects received professional tooth cleaning (plaque score = 0), a medium toothbrush to be used for tongue brushing, and asked to refrain from tooth cleaning and use of mouthwash

* Study 2 (7 days of restricted toothbrushing):
    Experimental groups (cross-over design):
    - Tongue brushing, supervised 2 x daily, 8 AM and 5 PM, 5 strokes per tongue quadrant, no dentifrice
    - Control: no tongue brushing

    Supervised toothbrushing 2 x daily for both groups using roll method and medium toothbrush; 5 strokes per tooth group, no dentifrice

    At baseline, all subjects received professional tooth cleaning (plaque score = 0), and instructions to refrain from other oral hygiene procedures

* Plaque extension over buccal surfaces of maxillary and mandibular canines and premolars determined using disclosing dye and standardized photography

* Analyses of mean plaque extension (% of buccal surface areas showing stained plaque)

Results:

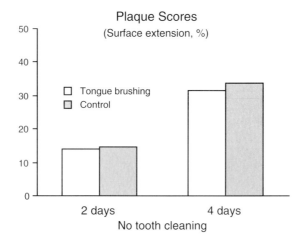

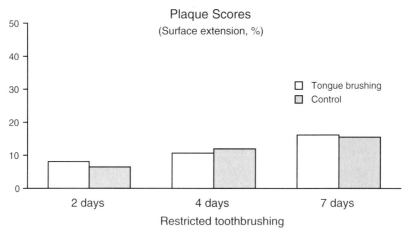

Comments:

- The extension of plaque over the buccal surfaces gradually increased in the subjects exposed to 4 days of no tooth cleaning. Tongue brushing did not seem to affect plaque formation.

- The plaque extension was more limited in the subjects exposed to restricted toothbrushing. Again, tongue brushing had no impact.

- These results, in limited numbers of dental hygiene students, deviate from those of Jacobson et al. (1973) and those of Study 1 by Gross et al. (1975) (pages 125-128). There is no apparent reason for these discrepancies of results, although it can not be excluded that the combination of tongue + palate brushing in the study by Jacobson et al. (1973) might have had some impact.

ROWLEY ET AL. (1987) studied plaque scores following tongue brushing and tongue scraping as a supplement to toothbrushing.

Subjects and procedures:

* 27 adults without periodontal involvement, without deeply fissured tongue, and not routinely practicing interdental cleaning or mechanical tongue cleaning

* 3 study groups (parallel design):
    - Tongue brushing, 10 strokes 2 x daily, without dentifrice using supplied toothbrush (N=9)
    - Tongue scraping, 10 strokes 2 x daily, without dentifrice using supplied tongue scraper (N=9)
    - Control: no tongue cleaning (N=9)

* Following baseline examination, all subjects received prophylaxis (plaque score = 0), a soft toothbrush and a standard toothpaste, asked to brush their teeth as normal and to refrain from use of other oral hygiene aids

* Plaque scores from buccal and lingual aspects of all teeth using disclosing dye and Turesky/Quigley-Hein index (scores 0-5)

* 2 weeks of observation

* Analyses of mean plaque scores

Results:

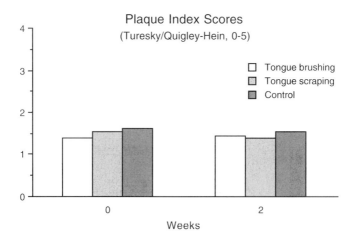

Comments:

- Baseline plaque scores, prior to prophylaxis, were similar for the 3 groups. After 2 weeks, plaque levels had returned to baseline levels. Supplementary tongue brushing or tongue scraping did not affect the plaque scores.

- The authors appropriately suggested that further studies should include more subjects per groups and subjects with greater baseline plaque scores.

- The results accord with those of Badersten et al. (1975) and those of Study 2 by Gross et al. (1975), but differ with those of Jacobson et al. (1973) and those of Study 1 by Gross et al. (1975). Again, there seems to be no obvious reason for these variations of results.

TONZETICH & NG (1976) studied the effect of tongue brushing and other cleansing procedures on early morning mouth odor.

Subjects and procedures:
* 8 nonsmoking males, 20-30 years of age, exhibiting objectional early morning mouth odor

* 4 consecutive tests, 1 week apart (cross-over design):
    - Toothbrushing during 2 minutes with a standard dentifrice
    - Tongue brushing during 2 minutes with a standard dentifrice
    - Toothbrushing + tongue brushing during 2 minutes with a standard dentifrice
    - Control: no cleansing

* Subjects abstained from oral hygiene, liquid and food in mornings prior to days of test

* Levels of hydrogen sulfide and methyl mercaptan (main volatile odorous substances in the oral cavity) measured by gas chromatography in samples of mouth air immediately prior to, and 30 and 60 minutes following test procedures[†]

* Analyses of mean concentrations of hydrogen sulfide and methyl mercaptan

[†] See Section 14: Mouthrinses: Effects on Oral Malodor, page 225, for methods of assessing mouth odor.

Results:

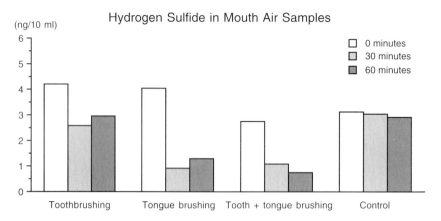

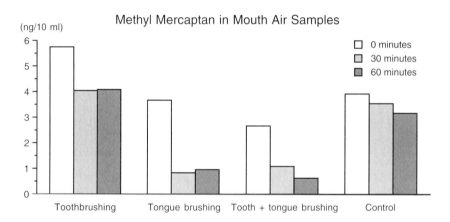

Comments:

- The pre-experimental concentrations of hydrogen sulfide and methyl mercaptan varied widely between the 4 test in this study, having a limited number of individuals. Nevertheless, the results suggest that tongue brushing is more effective in reducing early morning mouth odor than toothbrushing.

- Kaizu et al. (1978) compared the duration of reduction of methyl mercaptan levels in samples of mouth air following tongue scraping, toothbrushing, and rinsing with water in subjects with malodor. Reductions following tongue scraping lasted for about 100 minutes, whilst reductions following toothbrushing and rinsing only lasted for about 25 minutes.

- Bosy et al. (1994) studied the effects of a combination of tongue brushing and rinses with chlorhexidine on oral malodor. This study is reviewed in Section 14: Mouthrinses: Effects on Oral Malodor, pages 236-237.

Tongue brushing

Concluding remarks

Results of studies on tongue brushing as an adjunct to toothbrushing in order to reduce plaque levels are inconclusive.

The microorganisms able to adhere and multiply to the dorsum of the tongue may largely be different from those forming dental plaque. Accordingly, one may not expect that tongue brushing should be a significant adjunct to tooth-brushing for plaque preventive purposes.

For further research on tongue cleaning relative to plaque formation, it might be of value to assess plaque formation during periods without tooth cleaning longer than 2-4 days, and include analyses of the components of both tongue and plaque microbiota following tongue cleaning versus no tongue cleaning. In addition, study groups should be matched for the degree of coating/bacterial accumulation on the tongue, and possibly also limited to subjects with heavy tongue accumulations.

Tongue cleaning relative to mouth odor appears to be a field in need of additional research.

There seems to be no information available on the possibility of side effects from regular tongue cleaning.

Tongue brushing

References

Badersten, A., Egelberg, J., Jönsson, G. & Kroneng, M. (1975) Effect of tongue brushing on formation of dental plaque. Journal of Periodontology 46, 625-627.

Gross, A., Barnes, G.P. & Lyon, T.C. (1975) Effect of tongue brushing on tongue coating and dental plaque scores. Journal of Dental Research 54, 1236.

Jacobson, S.E., Crawford, J.J. & McFall, W.R. (1973) Oral physiotherapy of the tongue and palate: relationship to plaque control. Journal of the American Dental Association 87, 134-139.

Kaizu, T., Tsunoda, M., Aoki, H. & Kimura, K. (1978) Analysis of volatile sulphur compounds in mouth air by gas chromatography. Bulletin of Tokyo Dental College 19, 43-52.

Rowley, E.J., Schuchman, L.C., Tishk, M.N. & Carlson, H.C. (1987) Tongue brushing versus tongue scraping. A comparison of plaque reaccumulation, gingivitis and patient acceptance. Clinical Preventive Dentistry 9, 13-16.

Tonzetich, J. & Ng, S.K. (1976) Reduction of malodor by oral cleansing procedures. Oral Surgery, Oral Medicine, and Oral Pathology 42, 172-181.

SECTION 9

Dentifrices: Effects on plaque and gingivitis

Dentifrices are available on the market with claims of reducing plaque formation and gingivitis. The antimicrobial agents/formulae include:

- Triclosan combined with the copolymer polyvinylmethyl ether/maleic acid (PVM/MA). The copolymer is added for the purpose of enhancing the uptake of triclosan to tooth and mucosal surfaces (Colgate Paradent, Colgate Gum Protection, Colgate Total).

- Triclosan combined with zinc citrate (Mentadent, Mentadent P, Neo Mentadent P, Pepsodent Gum Health, Pepsodent Ultra).

- Sanguinarine combined with zinc chloride (PerioGard Veadent, Viadent).

- Stabilized stannous fluoride (Crest Gum Care, Crest Plus Gum Care).

Sanguinarine/zinc chloride dentifrices have primarily been evaluated following combined use with sanguinarine/zinc chloride mouthrinse. An example of results from this combined use is given in Section 13: Mouthrinses: Effects on Plaque and Gingivitis, pages 216-218.

Five trials representing the other antimicrobial agents/formulae above are selected for review in this section.

STUDIES PRESENTED IN THIS SECTION

Authors	Page	Subjects	Dentifrices	Observation interval
Lindhe et al. (1993)	139	Adults with plaque and gingivitis	Triclosan/copolymer Control	6 months
McClanahan et al. (1997)	143	Adults with plaque and gingivitis	Triclosan/copolymer Stannous fluoride Control	6 months
Svatun & Saxton (1993b)	146	Adults with plaque and gingivitis	Triclosan/copolymer Triclosan/zinc citrate Triclosan/pyrophosphate Control	7 months
Palomo et al. (1994)	149	Adults with plaque and gingivitis	Triclosan/copolymer Triclosan/zinc citrate Triclosan/pyrophosphate Control	6 months
Owens et al. (1997)	152	Adults with plaque and gingivitis	Triclosan/copolymer Triclosan/zinc citrate Stannous fluoride Control	18 weeks

LINDHE ET AL. (1993) compared the effects of a triclosan/copolymer dentifrice to a regular fluoride dentifrice.

Subjects and procedures:
* 110 subjects, 20-45 years of age, with plaque and moderate gingivitis (details
  on any attachment loss/interdental papillary heights not provided)

* Study groups, matched for age, plaque and gingivitis (parallel design):
    - Triclosan/copolymer dentifrice: triclosan (0.3%) + PVM/MA (2.0%) +
      sodium fluoride (0.243%) in silica abrasive base (Colgate Gum
      Protection) (N=56)

    - Control dentifrice: sodium fluoride (0.243%) in silica abrasive base
      (N=54)

* Following baseline examination, subjects received a soft toothbrush and the
  assigned toothpaste, were instructed to brush their teeth 2 x daily for 1
  minute, and to cover the entire length of the brush head with dentifrice

* No baseline prophylaxis

* Plaque scores at 6 sites of each tooth using disclosing dye and Turesky/
  Quigley-Hein index (scores 0-5)

* Gingivitis scores at 6 locations of each tooth using Löe-Silness index (scores
  0-3)

* 6 months of observation

* Analyses of:
    - mean plaque and gingivitis scores
    - plaque-free and gingivitis-free sites (%)

Results:

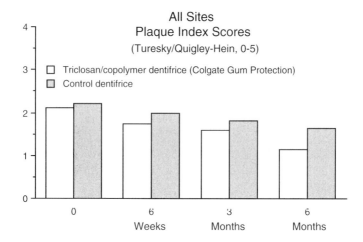

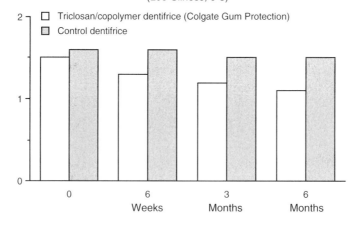

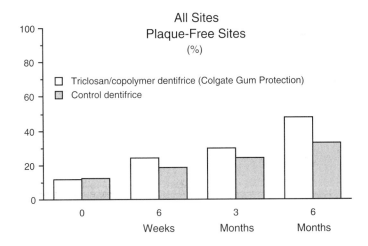

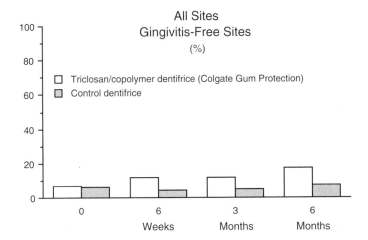

Comments:

- Mean plaque scores were gradually reduced for the control group during the 6-month observation period. The gingivitis scores for the control group, however, did not show a concomitant improvement. The improvement of the plaque scores would seem to be explained by the 'participation effect'.

- Mean plaque and gingivitis scores for the triclosan group improved beyond those for the control group.

- The proportions of plaque- and gingivitis-free sites for the triclosan group also improved beyond those for the control group.

- The triclosan dentifrice had a beneficial effect on mean plaque and gingivitis scores in all parts of the dentition, including posterior teeth and proximal sites (data not shown here). Data for the proportions of plaque- and gingivitis-free proximal sites would have been of interest.

- The magnitude of benefit for the triclosan/copolymer dentifrice as observed in this study may have some clinical significance.

- The results of this study are supported by findings of several other trials comparing triclosan dentifrices to control dentifrices (see review by Volpe et al. 1996).

McCLANAHAN ET AL. (1997) compared the effects of a triclosan/copolymer dentifrice, a stannous fluoride dentifrice and a regular fluoride dentifrice.

Subjects and procedures:

* 483 subjects, 19-70 years of age, with signs of gingivitis without having advanced periodontitis (details on any attachment loss/interdental papillary heights not provided)

* Initial prophylaxis followed by a 3-month pre-experimental period when all subjects were instructed to brush with a sodium fluoride/silica dentifrice

* Study groups, matched for sex and initial gingivitis (parallel design):
    - Triclosan/copolymer dentifrice: triclosan (0.3%) + PVM/MA (2.0%) + sodium fluoride (0.243%) in silica abrasive base (Colgate Gum Protection) (N=155)

    - Stabilized stannous fluoride dentifrice: stannous fluoride (0.454%) stabilized with sodium gluconate and stannous chloride in silica abrasive base (Crest Plus Gum Care) (N=154)

    - Control dentifrice: sodium fluoride (0.243%) in silica abrasive base (Crest Regular) (N=174)

* Following baseline examination, subjects received a 2nd prophylaxis, the assigned toothpaste, and were instructed to brush their teeth 2 x daily for at least 1 minute using their own toothbrushes

* Plaque scores at buccal and lingual aspects of each tooth using disclosing dye and Turesky/Quigley-Hein index (scores 0-5)

* Gingivitis scores at 6 locations of each tooth using Löe-Silness index (scores 0-3)

* Scores of extrinsic dental stain at buccal and lingual surfaces of all teeth using Meckel index; composite index of stain intensity (scores 0-3) multiplied by stain area (estimated to the nearest 5%)

* 6 months of observation

* Analyses of mean plaque, gingivitis and stain scores

Results:

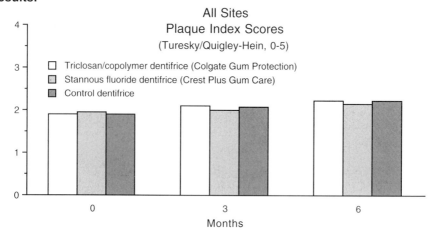

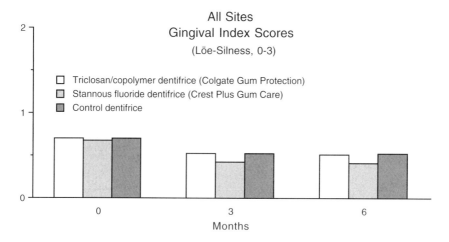

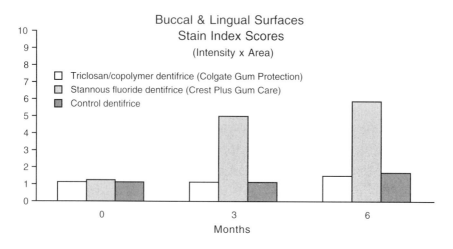

Comments:

- Plaque scores remained similar to the baseline scores (prior to 2nd prophylaxis) for all 3 study groups at both 3 and 6 months.

- Gingivitis scores were reduced at 3 and 6 months compared to baseline. Scores for the stannous fluoride dentifrice at 3 and 6 months were slightly lower than those for the triclosan and regular fluoride dentifrices.

- The fact that an initial prophylaxis was given 3 months prior to baseline should lessen the possibility that the reduction of gingivitis scores after 3 months of observation was caused by the 2nd prophylaxis. The decreased gingivitis scores for all 3 study groups after 3 and 6 months are somewhat unexpected in the light of the unaltered plaque scores. Results of examiner drift?

- Separate data for proximal sites were not presented.

- Significantly more dental stain was formed from use of stannous fluoride dentifrice than from use of triclosan and control dentifrices.

- Stannous fluoride dentifrices were compared to regular sodium fluoride dentifrices in 6-month studies by Beiswanger et al. (1995, 1997) and by Perlich et al. (1995). As for the study reviewed above, both of these studies showed similar plaque scores for test and control but slightly lower gingivitis scores for the stannous fluoride dentifrices. In addition, both of these studies also demonstrated more dental stain formed from use of stannous fluoride dentifrices than from use of regular fluoride dentifrices.

- In this trial, contradictory to the results by Lindhe et al. (1993) (pages 139-142), any plaque and gingivitis benefits for the triclosan/copolymer dentifrice as compared to a regular fluoride dentifrice were not observed.

- The authors stated that "evaluation of the oral mucosa at the three- and six-month examinations revealed no unexpected nor clinically significant mucosal effects associated with the use of test dentifrices".

SVATUN & SAXTON (1993b) compared the effects of a triclosan/copolymer dentifrice, a triclosan/zinc citrate dentifrice, a triclosan/pyrophosphate dentifrice and a regular fluoride dentifrice.

Subjects and procedures:

* 185 subjects, 19-44 years of age, with mild to moderate gingivitis without having periodontal pockets ≥5 mm (details on any attachment loss/interdental papillary heights not provided)

* Study groups, matched for gingival bleeding and calculus scores (parallel design):
    - Triclosan/copolymer dentifrice: triclosan (0.3%) + PVM/MA (2.0%) + sodium fluoride (0.243%) in silica abrasive base (Colgate Gum Protection) (N=46)

    - Triclosan/zinc citrate dentifrice: triclosan (0.3%) + zinc citrate (0.75%) + sodium monofluorophosphate (0.8%) in silica abrasive base (Mentadent) (N=46)

    - Triclosan/pyrophosphate dentifrice: triclosan (0.3%) + pyrophosphate (5.0%) + sodium fluoride (0.32%) in silica abrasive base (Crest Ultra Protection) (N=45)

    - Control dentifrice: sodium monofluorophosphate (0.8%) in silica abrasive base (N=48)

* Following prophylaxis and a short oral hygiene instruction at baseline, subjects received a soft toothbrush and the assigned toothpaste, and were instructed to brush their teeth 2 x daily

* Plaque scores at 3 sites of each tooth (buccal, mesial and lingual) using Silness-Löe index (scores 0-3)

* Bleeding following sulcular probing recorded at 3 locations of each tooth (buccal, mesial and lingual; presence/absence)

* 7 months of observation

* Analyses of:
    - mean plaque scores
    - % sites with bleeding on probing

Results:

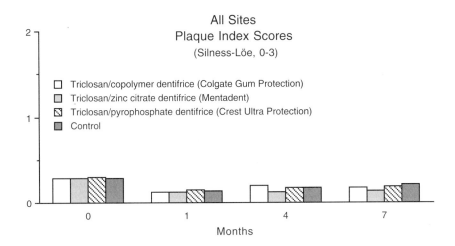

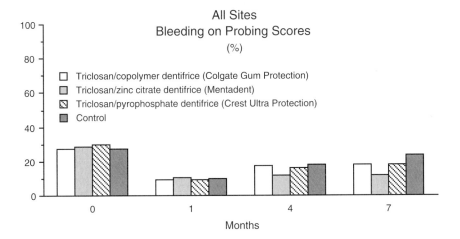

Comments:

- The participants of this study had comparatively low baseline plaque scores, which were further reduced after 1 month. Little difference in plaque scores was noted between dentifrice groups throughout the 7-month observation interval.

- Baseline bleeding on probing scores were also relatively low, but were further reduced 1 month following baseline prophylaxis and oral hygiene instruction. Subsequently, bleeding scores rebounded, most discernible for the control dentifrice, and least discernible for the triclosan/zinc citrate dentifrice.

- Studies on effects of oral hygiene procedures most often use records of plaque and gingivitis for 6 sites of each tooth: buccal + lingual + 4 proximal sites. In this study only 3 sites have been scored: buccal + lingual + mesial (= mesio-buccal?). This means that the data for all sites in this study have a 1/3 representation by proximal sites, as opposed a 2/3 representation in other studies. This may, at least in part, explain the comparatively low plaque and gingival index scores in this study. Separate presentation of results for the mesial sites would have been of value.

- The authors stated that "no adverse reactions of any kind were observed by the clinical examiner when assessing the subjects' hard and soft oral tissues; neither were side effects reported by any of the subjects during the study".

- The results of this study are supported by results of several other studies comparing triclosan/zinc citrate to control dentifrices by the same research group (Svatun & Saxton 1993a, Svatun et al. 1989a, 1989b, 1990).

- In this trial, little benefits were observed for the triclosan/copolymer and triclosan/pyrophosphate dentifrices as compared to a regular fluoride dentifrice.

PALOMO ET AL. (1994) compared the effects of a triclosan/copolymer dentifrice, a triclosan/zinc citrate dentifrice, a triclosan/pyrophosphate dentifrice and a regular fluoride dentifrice.

Subjects and procedures:
* 180 subjects, 18-65 years of age, with plaque and gingivitis (details on any attachment loss/interdental papillary heights not provided)

* Study groups, matched for plaque and gingivitis scores (parallel design):
    - Triclosan/copolymer dentifrice: triclosan (0.3%) + PVM/MA (2.0%) + sodium fluoride (0.243%) in silica abrasive base (Colgate Gum Protection) (N=42)

    - Triclosan/zinc citrate dentifrice: triclosan (0.2%) + zinc citrate (0.5%) + sodium monofluorophosphate (0.85%) in alumina abrasive base (Neo Mentadent P) (N=47)

    - Triclosan/pyrophosphate dentifrice: triclosan (0.3%) + pyrophosphate (5.0%) + sodium fluoride (0.32%) in silica abrasive base (Crest Ultra Protection) (N=47)

    - Control dentifrice: sodium fluoride (0.243%) in silica abrasive base (N=44)

* Following baseline examination, subjects received prophylaxis, a soft toothbrush and the assigned toothpaste, and were instructed to brush their teeth 2 x daily for 1 minute

* Plaque scores at 6 sites of each tooth using disclosing dye and Turesky/ Quigley-Hein index (scores 0-5)

* Gingivitis scores at 6 locations of each tooth using Löe-Silness index (scores 0-3)

* 6 months of observation

* Analyses of mean plaque and gingivitis scores

Results:

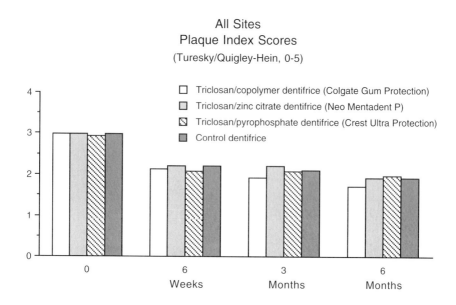

All Sites
Plaque Index Scores
(Turesky/Quigley-Hein, 0-5)

☐ Triclosan/copolymer dentifrice (Colgate Gum Protection)
▨ Triclosan/zinc citrate dentifrice (Neo Mentadent P)
▧ Triclosan/pyrophosphate dentifrice (Crest Ultra Protection)
▩ Control dentifrice

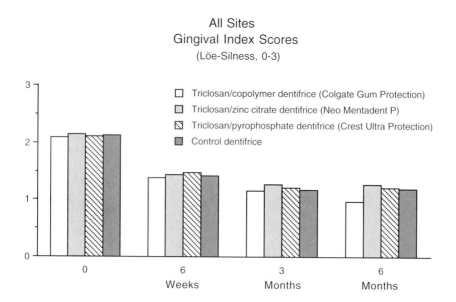

All Sites
Gingival Index Scores
(Löe-Silness, 0-3)

☐ Triclosan/copolymer dentifrice (Colgate Gum Protection)
▨ Triclosan/zinc citrate dentifrice (Neo Mentadent P)
▧ Triclosan/pyrophosphate dentifrice (Crest Ultra Protection)
▩ Control dentifrice

Comments:

- Baseline plaque scores and particularly baseline gingivitis scores were high for these participating individuals (note that the scale for the graph on gingival index scores on the previous page is different from that of the corresponding graphs on pages 140, 144 and 153 of this section).

- Plaque and gingivitis scores were notably reduced for all groups at 6 weeks compared to baseline (effect of baseline prophylaxis?). Additional improvement during the remainder of the 6-month study occurred primarily for the gingivitis scores. Results for the triclosan/copolymer dentifrice were somewhat better than those for the other dentifrices.

- Separate results for proximal sites were not given.

- In this trial, no benefits were observed for the triclosan/zinc citrate and triclosan/pyrophosphate dentifrices as compared to the control dentifrice.

- The authors stated that "no adverse effects were observed or reported".

OWENS ET AL. (1997) compared the effects of a triclosan/copolymer dentifrice, a triclosan/zinc citrate dentifrice, a stannous fluoride dentifrice and a regular fluoride dentifrice.

Subjects and procedures:

* 141 subjects, 18-65 years of age, with plaque and gingivitis without having untreated periodontitis requiring prompt treatment (details on any attachment loss/interdental papillary heights not provided)

* Study groups, matched for sex (parallel design):
  - Triclosan/copolymer dentifrice: triclosan (0.3%) + PVM/MA (2.0%) + sodium fluoride (0.32%) in silica abrasive base (Colgate Total) (N=36)

  - Triclosan/zinc citrate dentifrice: triclosan (0.3%) + zinc citrate (0.75%) + sodium fluoride (0.8%) in silica abrasive base (Mentadent P) (N=36)

  - Stabilized stannous fluoride dentifrice: stannous fluoride (0.454%) stabilized with sodium gluconate and stannous chloride in silica abrasive base (Crest Gum Care) (N=35)

  - Control dentifrice: sodium fluoride (0.1%) + monofluorophosphate (0.76%) in silica abrasive base (Colgate Regular) (N=34)

* Following baseline examination, subjects received prophylaxis, a multitufted toothbrush and the assigned toothpaste, and were instructed to brush their teeth 2 x daily

* Plaque scores at buccal and lingual aspects of each tooth using disclosing dye and Turesky/Quigley-Hein index (scores 0-5)

* Gingivitis scores at 6 locations of each tooth using Löe-Silness index (scores 0-3)

* 18 weeks of observation

* Analyses of mean plaque and gingivitis scores

Results:

All Sites
Plaque Index Scores
(Turesky/Quigley-Hein, 0-5)

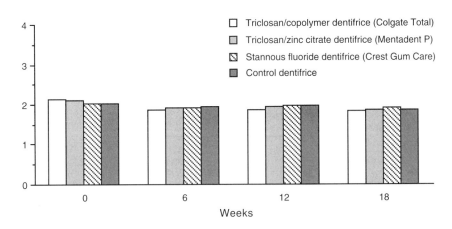

☐ Triclosan/copolymer dentifrice (Colgate Total)
▨ Triclosan/zinc citrate dentifrice (Mentadent P)
▨ Stannous fluoride dentifrice (Crest Gum Care)
▨ Control dentifrice

All Sites
Gingival Index Scores
(Löe-Silness, 0-3)

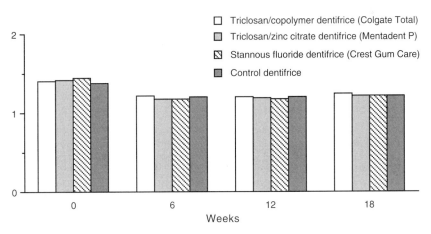

☐ Triclosan/copolymer dentifrice (Colgate Total)
▨ Triclosan/zinc citrate dentifrice (Mentadent P)
▨ Stannous fluoride dentifrice (Crest Gum Care)
▨ Control dentifrice

Comments:

- Plaque scores remained similar to the baseline scores (prior to prophylaxis) for all 4 study groups throughout the 18 weeks of observation.

- Gingivitis scores were reduced for all groups at 6 weeks compared to baseline and remained at this level throughout the study period. This reduction could be related to the prophylaxis at baseline.

- Thus, this study observed no differences between any of the antiplaque/anti-gingivitis dentifrices and the regular fluoride dentifrice. In another study, having 3 months of observation, the same group of researchers neither found any difference between a triclosan/copolymer dentifrice (Colgate Total) and 3 regular fluoride dentifrices (Binney et al. 1996).

Dentifrices: Effects on plaque and gingivitis

Concluding remarks

Results of recent research on antiplaque/antigingivitis dentifrices may be summarized as follows:

- Triclosan/copolymer dentifrices have been found to possess beneficial plaque and gingivitis effects as compared to regular fluoride dentifrices - illustrated by the results of Lindhe et al. (1993) reviewed above - and supported by results of several other studies (see review by Volpe et al. 1996).

- Triclosan/zinc citrate dentifrices have also been found to reduce plaque formation and gingivitis as compared to regular fluoride dentifrices - illustrated by the results of Svatun et al. (1993b) reviewed above - and supported by results of several other studies (Stephen et al. 1990, Svatun et al. 1989a, 1989b, 1990, Svatun & Saxton 1993a).

- Stannous fluoride dentifrices, likewise, have been found to have antigingivitis effects as compared to regular fluoride dentifrices - illustrated by the results of McClanahan et al. (1993) reviewed above - and supported by results of Beiswanger et al. (1995, 1997) and Perlich et al. (1995).

- When observed, the differences of results in favor of the antiplaque/antigingivitis dentifrices have generally been of modest or limited magnitude.

- Contradictory results with respect to superiority are available from studies comparing different antiplaque/antigingivitis dentifrices. Thus, Palomo et al. (1994) found a triclosan/copolymer dentifrice somewhat more effective in controlling plaque and gingivitis than a triclosan/zinc citrate dentifrice. Svatun & Saxton (1993b), on the other hand, observed a reversed superiority between these dentifrices, whilst Conforti et al. (1994) found no differences.

- As illustrated by results of Palomo et al. (1994), McClanahan et al. (1997) and Owens et al. (1997) reviewed above, studies have also failed to find any beneficial effects of antiplaque/antigingivitis dentifrices compared to regular fluoride dentifrices (also Binney et al. 1996).

- The antiplaque/antigingivitis effects of a dentifrice with various herbal extracts and with sodium bicarbonate as abrasive (Parodontax) have been evaluated in a couple of recent studies (not reviewed here). Yankell et al. (1993), using 6 months of observation, observed slightly lower plaque scores following use of Parodontax compared to a placebo dentifrice. However, this difference was not coupled with a difference in gingivitis scores. Mullally et al. (1995), using 6 weeks of observation, observed similar changes of both plaque and gingivitis scores following use of Parodontax and a control dentifrice.

In summary, it would seem that there is no dentifrice yet marketed with clinically significant or unquestioned beneficial effects on plaque formation and gingivitis.

As mentioned before, many studies on effectiveness or oral hygiene methods would have been easier to interpret, if:
- Subjects and sites to be included had been carefully selected with respect to intact versus reduced interdental papillary height;
- Data on % plaque-free and % gingivitis-free proximal/interdental sites had been presented.

Use of the specially formulated dentifrices during periods of 6-12 months does not seem to induce any adverse effects on the oral mucosa. (Also, see Section 11: Dentifrices: Effects on Supragingival Calculus, pages 169-181).

The oral microflora has been evaluated following use of triclosan/copolymer dentifrices for periods of 6-12 months. Neither shifts of the flora, nor development of resistant strains have been discovered (see review by Volpe et al. 1996). Although less investigated, these negative findings may also hold true for triclosan/zinc citrate dentifrices (Jones et al. 1988, Stephen et al. 1990, Renvert & Birkhed 1995).

Dentifrices: Effects on plaque and gingivitis

References

Beiswanger, B.B., Doyle, P.M., Jackson, R.D., Mallatt, M.E., Mau, M.S., Bollmer, B.W., Crisanti, M.M., Guay, C.B., Lanzalaco, A.C., Lukacovic, M.F., Majeti, S. & McClanahan, S.F. (1995) The clinical effect of dentifrices containing stabilized stannous fluoride on plaque formation and gingivitis - A six-month study with *ad libitum* brushing. Journal of Clinical Dentistry 6 (spec. issue), 46-53.

Beiswanger, B.B., McClanahan, S.F., Bartizek, R.D., Lanzalaco, A.C., Bacca, L.A. & White, D.J. (1997) The comparative efficacy of stabilized stannous fluoride dentifrice, peroxide/baking soda dentifrice and essential oil mouthrinse for the prevention of gingivitis. Journal of Clinical Dentistry 8, 46-53.

Binney, A., Addy, M., Owens, J., Faulkner, J., McKeown, S. & Everatt, L. (1996) A 3-month home use study comparing the oral hygiene and gingival health benefits of triclosan and conventional fluoride toothpastes. Journal of Clinical Periodontology 23, 1020-1024.

Conforti, N.J., Smith, I., Davies, R., Proskin, H., Chaknis, P., DeVizio, W., Petrone, M., Volpe, A. & McCool, J.J. (1994) Comparative efficacy of two commercially available dentifrices containing triclosan in the control of plaque and gingivitis: A six-month clinical study in Scotland. Journal of Clinical Dentistry 5, 70-73.

Jones, C.L., Ritchie, J.A., Marsh, P.D. & van der Ouderaa, F. (1988) The effect of long-term use of a dentifrice containing zinc citrate and a non-ionic agent on the oral flora. Journal of Dental Research 67, 46-50.

Lindhe, J., Rosling, B., Socransky, S.S. & Volpe, A.R., (1993) The effect of a triclosan-containing dentifrice on established plaque and gingivitis. Journal of Clinical Periodontology 20, 327-334.

McClanahan, S.F., Beiswanger, B.B., Bartizek, R.D., Lanzalaco, A.C., Bacca, L. & White, D.J. (1997) A comparison of stabilized stannous fluoride dentifrice and triclosan/copolymer dentifrice for efficacy in the reduction of gingivitis and gingival bleeding: Six-month clinical results. Journal of Clinical Dentistry 8, 39-45.

Mullally, B.H., James, J.A., Coulter, W.A. & Linden, G.J. (1995) The efficacy of a herbal-based toothpaste on the control of plaque and gingivitis. Journal of Clinical Periodontology 22, 686-689.

Owens, J., Addy, M. & Faulkner, J. (1997) An 18-week home-use study comparing the oral hygiene and gingival health benefits of triclosan and fluoride toothpastes. Journal of Clinical Periodontology 24, 626-631.

Palomo, F., Wantland, L., Sanchez, A., Volpe, A.R., McCool, J. & DeVizio, W. (1994) The effect of three commercially available dentifrices containing triclosan on supragingival plaque formation and gingivitis: A six month clinical study. International Dental Journal 44, 75-81.

Perlich, M.A., Bacca, L.A., Bollmer, B.W., Lanzalaco, A.C., McClanahan, S.F., Sewak, L.K., Beiswanger, B.B., Eichold, W.A., Hull, J.R., Jackson, R.D. & Mau, M.S. (1995) The clinical effect of a stabilized stannous fluoride dentifrice on plaque formation, gingivitis and gingival bleeding: A six-month study. Journal of Clinical Dentistry 6 (spec. issue), 54-58.

Renvert, S. & Birkhed, D. (1995) Comparison between 3 triclosan dentifrices on plaque, gingivitis and salivary microflora. Journal of Clinical Periodontology 22, 63-70.

Stephen, K.W., Saxton, C.A., Jones, C.L., Ritchie, J.A. & Morrison, T. (1990) Control of gingivitis and calculus by a dentifrice containing zinc salt and triclosan. Journal of Periodontology 61, 674-679.

Svatun, B. & Saxton, C.A. (1993a) The effects of a silica dentifrice containing triclosan and zinc citrate on supragingival plaque and calculus formation and the control of gingivitis. International Dental Journal 43, 431-439.

Svatun, B. & Saxton, C.A. (1993b) The effects of three silica dentifrices containing triclosan on supragingival plaque and calculus formation and on gingivitis. International Dental Journal 43, 441-452.

Svatun, B., Saxton, C.A., Rölla, G. & van der Ouderaa, F. (1989a) A 1-year study on the maintenance of gingival health by a dentifrice containing a zinc salt and a non-anionic antimicrobial agent. Journal of Clinical Periodontology 16, 75-80.

Svatun, B., Saxton, C.A., Rölla, G. & van der Ouderaa, F. (1989b) One-year study of the efficacy of a dentifrice containing zinc citrate and triclosan to maintain gingival health. Scandinavian Journal of Dental Research 97, 242-246.

Svatun, B., Saxton, C.A. & Rölla, G. (1990) Six-month study of the effect of a dentifrice containing zinc citrate and triclosan on plaque, gingival health, and calculus. Scandinavian Journal of Dental Research 98, 301-304.

Volpe, A.R., Petrone, M.E., DeVizio, W., Davies, R.M. & Proskin, H.M. (1996) A review of plaque, gingivitis, calculus and caries clinical efficacy studies with a fluoride dentifrice containing triclosan and PVM/MA copolymer. Journal of Clinical Dentistry 7 (suppl.) S1-S14.

Yankell, S.L., Emling, R.C. & Perez, B. (1993) Six-month evaluation of Parodontax dentifrice compared to a placebo dentifrice. Journal of Clinical Dentistry 4, 26-30.

Dentifrices: Effects on periodontitis

The effects of daily use of a triclosan/copolymer dentifrice (Colgate Total) on progression of periodontitis have been investigated in 2 recent 3-year trials. Both of these studies are reviewed.

STUDIES PRESENTED IN THIS SECTION

Authors	Page	Subjects	Dentifrices	Observation interval
Ellwood et al. (1998)	161	11-13 year-olds	Triclosan/copolymer Control	3 years
Rosling et al. (1997a)	163	Advanced periodontitis patients on maintenance	Triclosan/copolymer Control	3 years

ELLWOOD ET AL. (1998) compared the effects of a triclosan/copolymer dentifrice to a control dentifrice on progression of periodontitis during 3 years in adolescents.

Subjects and procedures:
* 480 adolescents, 11-13 years of age, from 6 different local schools (63% European origin, 36% Asian origin)

* Study groups, matched for school, ethnic group and sex (parallel design):
  - Triclosan/copolymer dentifrice: triclosan (0.3%) + PVM/MA (2.0%) + sodium fluoride (0.243%) in silica abrasive base (Colgate Total) (N=239)

  - Control dentifrice: sodium fluoride (0.243%) in silica abrasive base (N=241)

* Following baseline examination, subjects received assigned toothpaste and a toothbrush, and were instructed to brush their teeth 2 x daily; new toothpaste + toothbrush mailed every 8th week

* Periodontal attachment loss measured by identifying the cemento-enamel junction (CEJ) and measuring the distance to the base of probing depth ('pocket') using a periodontal probe:
$$0 = \text{no attachment loss, CEJ not probeable}$$
$$>0 = \text{CEJ probeable, but distance to base of pocket less than 1 mm}$$
$$\geq 1 = \text{distance to base of pocket 1 mm or more}$$

* Recordings at mesio-buccal and disto-buccal sites of all 1st molars, maxillary left 1st and 2nd incisors, and mandibular right 1st and 2nd incisors (total of 8 teeth and 16 sites)

* 3 years of observation

* Analyses of % subjects with ≥ 1 sites with attachment loss >0 mm and ≥ 1 mm

Results:

% Subjects Showing ≥1 Sites with Probing Attachment Loss of Different Magnitude between Baseline and 3-year Examinations

Magnitude of change	Triclosan/copolymer dentifrice		Control dentifrice	
	Baseline	3 years	Baseline	3 years
>0 mm	2	23	3	25
≥1 mm	2	13	3	15

Comments:

- During the 3 years of observation there was an increase in % individuals with probing attachment loss for ≥1 of the investigated 18 sites. This increase was similar for both study groups.

- In their data analysis, the authors also calculated the mean probing attachment loss over the 3 years for subgroups of individuals. For the subgroup of those 25% of all subjects that showed the deepest mean probing depth at baseline, statistically significantly less probing attachment loss was found for individuals using the triclosan/copolymer dentifrice than for individuals using the control dentifrice: a mean of 0.07 mm as compared to a mean of 0.13 mm.

- The above limited difference between test and control subjects (0.06 mm) motivated the authors to conclude that "In the upper quartile of participants with the deepest periodontal pockets at baseline the mean increment of attachment loss over the three years was 50% less in the test group than the control group."

- The proportions of subjects having ≥1 sites with probing attachment loss >0 mm and ≥1 mm were not reported for the above subgroup (as they were for the entire study groups, see table above). Such numbers would have been more clinically meaningful than the minute difference of mean values.

- The authors also recorded plaque and bleeding on probing scores. These scores were presented for the baseline examination, but unfortunately not for the examinations carried out after 18 and 36 months.

- It was stated that "No adverse side-effects attributable to the use of either the control or test dentifrice were observed throughout the 3 year study".

ROSLING ET AL. (1997a) compared the effects of a triclosan/copolymer dentifrice to a control dentifrice on disease progression over 3 years in periodontitis patients on maintenance.

Subjects and procedures:

* 60 subjects, 34-67 years of age, previously provided nonsurgical therapy for advanced periodontal disease, having received maintenance treatment every 3rd month for 3-5 years, and with:
    - Average, radiographic proximal bone loss in the dentition >40%
    - Signs of deepened periodontal pockets and additional attachment loss during the 3-5 years of maintenance
    - ≥2 sites with probing depth ≥6 mm in each quadrant at study baseline

* Study groups, matched for mean probing depth (parallel design):
    - Triclosan/copolymer dentifrice: triclosan (0.3%) + PVM/MA (2.0%) + sodium fluoride (0.243%) in silica abrasive base (Colgate Total) (N=30)

    - Control dentifrice: sodium fluoride (0.243%) in silica abrasive base (N=30)

* Following baseline examination, subjects received assigned toothpaste and a Colgate Precision toothbrush, and "information how to brush their teeth in a proper way"

* Recalls every 3rd month for additional oral hygiene instruction as needed

* No professional subgingival therapy provided at the 3-month recalls

* Recordings at 6 sites of each tooth:
    - bleeding on probing (% sites with bleeding)
    - probing depths (mm)
    - probing attachment levels (mm), determined from fixed landmarks on individually fabricated stents

* 3 years of observation

* Analyses of:
    - mean bleeding scores, probing depths and probing attachment levels
    - frequency distribution of probing depths ≤3 mm, 4-5 mm and ≥6 mm
    - incidence of sites with probing attachment loss ≥2 mm

Results:

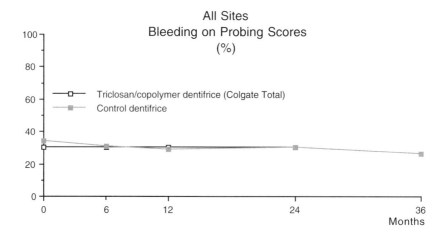

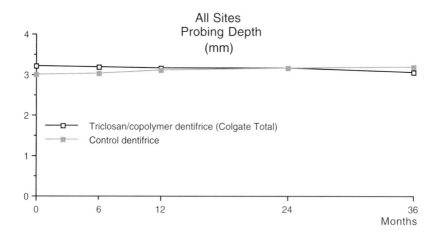

% Sites with Different Probing Depths at Baseline and 36-month Examinations

Probing depth	Triclosan/copolymer dentifrice			Control dentifrice		
	Baseline	36 months	Difference	Baseline	36 months	Difference
≤3 mm	57	61	+4	61	59	-2
4-5 mm	31	27	-4	28	28	0
≥6 mm	12	12	0	11	13	+2

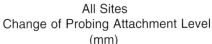

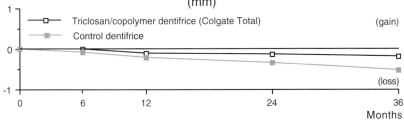

All Sites
Change of Probing Attachment Level
(mm)

% Sites with Probing Attachment Loss ≥2 mm between Baseline and 36-month Examinations for Sites with Different Baseline Probing Depth

Baseline probing depth	Triclosan/copolymer dentifrice		Control dentifrice	
	No loss	Loss	No loss	Loss
≤3 mm	95	5	90	10
4-5 mm	97	3	94	6
≥6 mm	99	1	96	4

Comments:

- Bleeding on probing scores remained unchanged for both study groups during the 3-year observation period.

- Mean probing depth tended to decrease for the triclosan/copolymer group and increase for the control group. The difference between the 2 groups in probing depth change from baseline to 3-year examinations (mean = 0.3 mm) was found to reach statistical significance.

- Calculations of the proportions of sites with probing depths ≤3 mm, 4-5 mm and ≥6 mm also indicated a tendency that probing depths improved more for the triclosan/copolymer group. Results of statistical analysis were not reported for these calculations.

- Some loss of mean probing attachment levels occurred for both groups. The loss for the control was slightly more than that for the triclosan/copolymer group. The difference between the groups reached statistical significance.

- The proportions of sites with probing attachment loss ≥2 mm also indicated a tendency that attachment levels deteriorated more for the triclosan/copolymer group. Result of statistical analysis for these calculations was not reported.

- A new set of radiographs were taken after 3 years. Compared to baseline, some loss of proximal bone levels was noted for both groups (mean for triclosan/copolymer group = 0.20 mm; mean for control group = 0.34 mm; difference between groups statistically significant).

- The results of this study, thus, indicate some benefits for the triclosan/copolymer dentifrice as compared to the control dentifrice with respect to periodontal disease progression. In the light of this difference, it is somewhat surprising that the bleeding scores showed no difference between the 2 groups.

- Plaque scores were not reported. However, in 20 subjects from each group, samples of the subgingival microflora were obtained with paper points from 4 sites and pooled (deepest probing depth in each quadrant). The mean number of bacteria sampled in this way indicated reductions after 3 years compared to baseline for both groups. Only the reduction for the triclosan/copolymer group was statistically significant (Rosling et al. 1997b).

- The proportions of smokers and nonsmokers in the 2 study groups were not reported.

Dentifrices: Effects on periodontitis

Concluding remarks

The undertaking of 3-year studies to investigate the possibility that dentifrices with antimicrobial agents might reduce periodontitis progression should be commended.

The results of the 2 available studies on use of the triclosan/copolymer dentifrice suggest that this dentifrice may retard progression of periodontitis as compared to a control dentifrice. These findings are somewhat remarkable since none of these 2 studies have demonstrated that the triclosan/copolymer dentifrice affected the degree of gingivitis.

Results of other studies investigating the effects of the triclosan/copolymer dentifrice on gingivitis have neither convincingly shown that this dentifrice affects gingivitis more than a control dentifrice (See Section 9: Dentifrices: Effects on Plaque and Gingivitis, pages 137-158).

The possibility that the triclosan/copolymer dentifrice somehow may affect the subgingival microbiota and thereby reduce periodontitis progression have some support from the results of Rosling et al. (1997b), but needs additional research.

More complete data presentation in the available studies on the triclosan/copolymer dentifrice would have been an advantage for their interpretation.

In summary, additional research seems required to allow any conclusions on the effects of dentifrices with triclosan/copolymer (or other antimicrobial agents) on progression of periodontitis.

Dentifrices: Effects on periodontitis

References

Ellwood, R.P., Worthington, H.V., Blinkhorn, A.S.B., Volpe, A.R., & Davies, R.M. (1998) Effect of triclosan/copolymer dentifrice on the incidence of periodontal attachment loss in adolescents. Journal of Clinical Periodontology 25, 363-367.

Rosling, B., Wannfors, B., Volpe, A.R., Furuichi, Y., Ramberg, P. & Lindhe, J. (1997a) The use of triclosan/copolymer dentifrice may retard the progression of periodontitis. Journal of Clinical Periodontology 24, 873-880.

Rosling, B., Dahlén, G., Volpe, A.R., Furuichi, Y., Ramberg, P. & Lindhe, J. (1997b) Effect of triclosan on the subgingival microbiota of periodontitis-susceptible subjects. Journal of Clinical Periodontology 24, 881-887.

SECTION 11

Dentifrices: Effects on supragingival calculus

Dentifrices with claims of reducing formation of supragingival calculus are available on the market. The anticalculus agents/formulae include:

- Triclosan/PVM/MA copolymer (Colgate Paradent, Colgate Gum Protection, Colgate Total).

- Triclosan/zinc citrate (Mentadent, Mentadent P, Pepsodent Ultra).

- Pyrophosphate (Crest Tartar Control).

- Pyrophosphate/PVM/MA copolymer (Colgate Tartar Control)

- Pyrophosphate/triclosan (Crest Gum Health, Crest Ultra Protection, Crest Complete).

It has been suggested that the anticalculus effect is caused by inhibition of nucleation and crystal growth of calcium phosphate mineral. This may delay mineralization of the plaque and make it more susceptible to mechanical removal. The capacity to inhibit crystal growth has been attributed to pyrophosphate, zinc citrate as well as the PVM/MA copolymer.

The anticalculus effect of toothpastes has been evaluated by measurements of calculus formation on the lingual aspects of the mandibular anterior teeth using the Volpe index: The height of the supragingival calculus is measured to the nearest half mm using a calibrated periodontal probe. A total of 18 measurements are taken; 3 lingual sites for each of the 6 mandibular teeth (mesio-lingual, mid-lingual, disto-lingual; recorded perpendicular to the gingival margin).

Four recent trials representing the anticalculus agents/formulae above are selected for review in this section.

STUDIES PRESENTED IN THIS SECTION

Authors	Page	Subjects	Dentifrices	Observation interval
White et al. (1996)	171	Adults prone to calculus formation	Pyrophosphate Pyrophosphate/copolymer Control	6 months
Fairbrother et al. (1997)	173	Adults prone to calculus formation	Pyrophosphate/triclosan Triclosan/copolymer Triclosan/zinc citrate Control	4 months
Volpe et al. (1992)	175	Adults prone to calculus formation	Pyrophosphate/triclosan Triclosan/copolymer Control	3 months
Bánóczy et al. (1995)	177	Adults prone to calculus formation	Pyrophosphate/copolymer Triclosan/copolymer Triclosan/zinc citrate Control	3 months

WHITE ET AL. (1996) compared the effects of a pyrophosphate dentifrice, a pyrophosphate/copolymer dentifrice and a regular fluoride dentifrice.

Subjects and procedures:

* 800 adults screened for tendency towards formation of supragingival calculus on lingual aspects of mandibular anterior teeth during a 3-month pre-experimental period; initiated with prophylaxis, using toothbrushing with a regular fluoride dentifrice, and no other oral hygiene products/measures

* 686 subjects accepted, having Volpe total calculus score ≥7 mm, (corresponding to an average calculus height per site of ≥0.4 mm); 653 of these subjects completed the study

* Study groups, matched for sex and pre-experimental calculus score (parallel design):
    - Pyrophosphate dentifrice: pyrophosphate (5.0%) + sodium fluoride (0.243%) in silica abrasive base (Crest Tartar Control) (N=218)

    - Pyrophosphate/copolymer dentifrice: pyrophosphate (1.3%) + PVM/MA (1.5%) + sodium fluoride (0.243%) in silica abrasive base (Colgate Tartar Control) (N=219)

    - Control dentifrice: sodium fluoride (0.243%) in silica abrasive base (Advanced Formula Crest) (N=216)

* Following a 2nd prophylaxis at baseline, subjects received a soft toothbrush and the assigned toothpaste, were instructed to brush their teeth 2 x daily for 1 minute and to cover the entire length of the brush head with dentifrice, and not to use any other oral hygiene products/measures

* Supragingival calculus recorded at 3 lingual sites of each of the 6 mandibular anterior teeth using Volpe index

* 6 months of observation

* Analyses of mean calculus scores (mm)

Results:

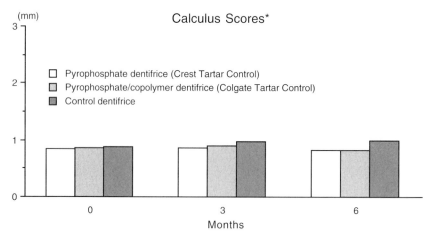

* The original data have been divided by 18 to provide the average calculus height per site in mm.

Comments:

- The participants of this study formed moderate amounts of supragingival calculus as determined from the 3-month pre-experimental period. At baseline, average heights of the calculus amounted to 0.8-0.9 mm.

- The amounts of calculus formed after 3 months for all 3 groups were similar to the amounts formed during the 3-month pre-experimental period.

- There was no additional growth in height of the calculus between 3 and 6 months.

- Slightly less calculus was formed using the pyrophosphate and the pyrophosphate/copolymer dentifrices than the regular fluoride dentifrice (statistically significant at both 3 and 6 months, 10% and 8% less respectively at 3 months; 17% and 17% less respectively at 6 months). However, considering the small differences, and also the similarity between the 3-month experimental scores and the 3-month pre-experimental scores, this study would not seem to demonstrate any clinically important benefits to the specially formulated toothpastes.

- The authors stated that "no serious or adverse effects related to product use were reported by either the subjects or the investigators".

FAIRBROTHER ET AL. (1997) compared the effects of a pyrophosphate/triclosan dentifrice, a triclosan/copolymer dentifrice, a triclosan/zinc citrate dentifrice and a regular fluoride dentifrice.

Subjects and procedures:

* 536 adult subjects with Volpe total calculus score ≥3 mm (corresponding to an average calculus height per site of ≥0.2 mm) as determined from a 3-month pre-experimental period initiated with prophylaxis and with use of a regular fluoride toothpaste 2 x daily

* Study groups, matched for age, sex and pre-experimental calculus score (parallel design):
    - Pyrophosphate/triclosan dentifrice: pyrophosphate (5.0%) + triclosan (0.28%) + sodium fluoride (0.145%) in silica abrasive base (Crest Complete) (N=134)

    - Triclosan/copolymer dentifrice: triclosan (0.3%) + PVM/MA (2.0%) + sodium fluoride (0.243%) in silica abrasive base (Colgate Total) (N=138)

    - Triclosan/zinc citrate dentifrice: triclosan (0.2%) + zinc citrate (0.5%) + sodium monofluorophosphate (0.15%) in silica abrasive base (Mentadent P) (N=129)

    - Control dentifrice: sodium fluoride (0.243%) in silica abrasive base (N=135)

* Following a 2nd prophylaxis at baseline, subjects received a toothbrush and the assigned toothpaste, and were instructed to brush their teeth 2 x daily

* Supragingival calculus recorded at 3 lingual sites of each of the 6 mandibular anterior teeth using Volpe index

* 4 months of observation

* Analyses of mean calculus scores (mm)

Results:

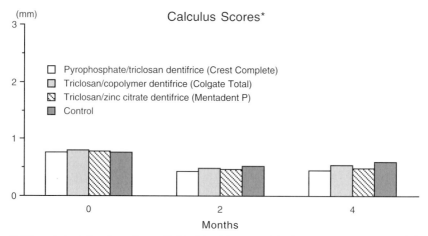

* The original data have been divided by 18 to provide the average calculus height
  per site in mm.

Comments:

- The participants of this study formed moderate amounts of supragingival calculus as determined from the 3-month pre-experimental period. Baseline
  average calculus height per site amounted to around 0.8 mm.

- There was little growth in height of the calculus between 2 and 4 months as
  reflected with the Volpe index.

- Surprisingly, less calculus was formed during 4-month use of the control
  dentifrice than during 3-month use of the same dentifrice pre-experimentally.

- The authors pointed out that the 4-month results showed a statistically significant reduction of calculus scores in mm compared to the control for the
  pyrophosphate/triclosan and triclosan/zinc citrate dentifrices (23% and 19%
  respectively), but not for the triclosan/copolymer toothpaste.

- The clinical importance of the benefits of the pyrophosphate/triclosan and
  triclosan/zinc citrate dentifrices is debatable, considering the minor differences observed.

- The authors stated that "no adverse events or effects on oral soft tissues
  related to product use were noted during the course of the trial".

VOLPE ET AL. (1992) compared the effects of a pyrophosphate/triclosan denti-frice, a triclosan/copolymer dentifrice and a regular fluoride dentifrice.

Subjects and procedures:
* 138 adult subjects prone to calculus formation as determined from a 3-month pre-experimental period initiated with prophylaxis, using toothbrushing with a regular fluoride dentifrice, and no other oral hygiene products/measures; no minimum calculus score reported

* Study groups, matched for pre-experimental calculus score (parallel design):
    - Pyrophosphate/triclosan dentifrice: pyrophosphate (5.0%) + triclosan (0.3%) + sodium fluoride (0.243%) in silica abrasive base (Crest Gum Health) (N=46)

    - Triclosan/copolymer dentifrice: triclosan (0.3%) + PVM/MA (2.0%) + sodium fluoride (0.243%) in silica abrasive base (Colgate Gum Protection) (N=47)

    - Control dentifrice: sodium fluoride (0.243%) in silica abrasive base (N=45)

* Following a 2nd prophylaxis at baseline, subjects received a soft toothbrush and the assigned toothpaste, were instructed to brush their teeth 2 x daily for 1 minute, and not to use any other oral hygiene products/measures

* Supragingival calculus recorded at 3 lingual sites of each of the 6 mandibular anterior teeth using Volpe index

* 3 months of observation

* Analyses of mean calculus scores (mm)

Results:

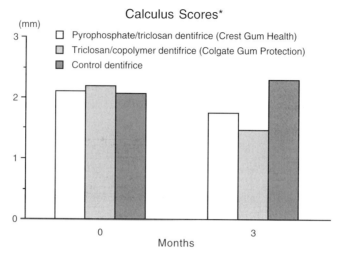

Calculus Scores*

(mm)

☐ Pyrophosphate/triclosan dentifrice (Crest Gum Health)
☐ Triclosan/copolymer dentifrice (Colgate Gum Protection)
■ Control dentifrice

Months

* The original data have been divided by 18 to provide the average calculus height per site in mm.

Comments:

- The participants selected for this study formed marked amounts of supragingival calculus. The baseline calculus heights per site after a 3-month pre-experimental period averaged around 2 mm.

- Results after 3 months showed reduced amounts of calculus for both the pyrophosphate/triclosan and triclosan/copolymer dentifrices as compared to the regular fluoride dentifrice (24% and 36% respectively). This degree of reduction in what appears to be heavy calculus formers may have clinical interest.

- The clinical benefits of the specially formulated toothpastes would have been easier to evaluate if data for % sites with presence/absence of calculus had been presented. Such data probably relate more to the efforts needed to remove the calculus.

- The authors stated that "there were no side effects of the hard and soft tissues of the oral cavity either observed by the examining dentist or reported by the subjects".

BÁNÓCZY ET AL. (1995) compared the effects of a pyrophosphate/copolymer dentifrice, a triclosan/copolymer dentifrice, a triclosan/zinc citrate dentifrice and a regular fluoride dentifrice.

Subjects and procedures:
* 143 adult subjects prone to calculus formation as determined from a 2-month pre-experimental period initiated with prophylaxis, using toothbrushing with a regular fluoride dentifrice, and no other oral hygiene products/measures; no minimum calculus score reported

* Study groups, matched for pre-experimental calculus score (parallel design):
  - Pyrophosphate/copolymer dentifrice: pyrophosphate (1.3%) + PVM/MA (1.5%) + sodium fluoride (0.243%) in silica abrasive base (Colgate Tartar Control) (N=35)

  - Triclosan/copolymer dentifrice: triclosan (0.3%) + PVM/MA (2.0%) + sodium fluoride (0.243%) in silica abrasive base (Colgate Total) (N=37)

  - Triclosan/zinc citrate dentifrice: triclosan (0.3%) + zinc citrate (0.75%) + sodium monofluorophosphate (1.14%) in silica abrasive base (Pepsodent Ultra) (N=35)

  - Control dentifrice: sodium fluoride (0.243%) in silica abrasive base (N=36)

* Following a 2nd prophylaxis at baseline, subjects received a soft toothbrush and the assigned toothpaste, and were instructed to brush their teeth 2 x daily for 1 minute

* Supragingival calculus recorded at 3 lingual sites of each of the 6 mandibular anterior teeth using Volpe index

* 3 months of observation

* Analyses of mean calculus scores (mm)

Results:

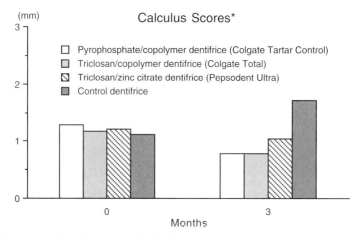

Calculus Scores*

* The original data have been divided by 18 to provide the average calculus height per site in mm.

Comments:

- The participants selected for this study formed notable amounts of supragingival calculus. The baseline average calculus heights after a 2-month pre-experimental period amounted to 1.2-1.3 mm.

- Results after 3 months showed reduced amounts of calculus for the pyrophosphate/copolymer, triclosan/copolymer and triclosan/zinc citrate dentifrices as compared to the regular fluoride dentifrice (55%, 55% and 39% respectively). This degree of reduction in what appears to be heavy calculus formers would seem to be of clinical interest.

- Again, the clinical benefits of the specially formulated toothpastes would have been easier to evaluate if data for % sites with presence/absence of calculus had been presented.

- The authors stated that "there were no adverse effects on the oral soft and hard tissues either reported or observed during the entire course of this study".

Dentifrices: Effects on supragingival calculus

Concluding remarks

A multitude of studies on anticalculus dentifrices has been published during recent years. Collectively, the results indicate that formation of supragingival calculus on the lingual aspects of mandibular anterior teeth can be affected by the use of such toothpastes. This would seem to include all the agents/formulae listed in the introduction of this section (page 169).

Results of trials on anticalculus dentifrices are characteristically tabulated using the total scores of the Volpe index (all 18 sites added). The differences compared to control dentifrices are expressed as % reduction of these scores, which typically varies between 15-50% and commonly amounts to 30-40% in trials of 3-6 months of duration (see review by Volpe et al. 1992). This corresponds to average reductions of the height of the calculus generally ranging between 0.1-0.5 mm. Obviously, the decrease in amount of calculus is a function of the efficacy of the dentifrice under study as well as the rate of calculus formation by the selected participants.

From a clinical perspective, anticalculus effects expressed as increases in % sites free of calculus - and in particular - increases in % subjects free of calculus would seem meaningful. It is unfortunate that such data are seldom provided in recent studies. In 2 less recent studies, however, data on sites and individuals free of calculus have also been presented, offering comparisons to the treatment effects as expressed by means.

Schiff (1987) compared a pyrophosphate dentifrice to a control dentifrice over 6 months and observed:
- reduction of mean calculus score = 36%;
- reduction of sites without calculus = 22%; and
- reduction of individuals without calculus = 15%.

Similarly, Lobene (1987) compared a pyrophosphate/copolymer dentifrice to a control dentifrice over 3 months and observed:
- reduction of mean calculus score = 50%;
- reduction of sites without calculus = 23%; and
- reduction of individuals without calculus = 15%.

Thus, it appears that the numbers on % improvement become less impressive if they are based upon calculus free sites and calculus free individuals.

The number of scaling strokes required to remove the calculus formed during the 6-month observation period was recorded by White et al. (1996) in their study (reviewed on pages 171-172). It was found that the reductions of the Volpe index scores observed for the anticalculus dentifrices as compared to the control dentifrice were coupled with corresponding decreases in strokes required to remove the calculus.

Gingivitis levels have not been recorded in studies on anticalculus dentifrices. Therefore, it is not known if the use of these dentifrices would be combined with any benefits relative to gingivitis/periodontitis. The advantages may primarily relate to some reductions in scaling efforts and some time saved during recall treatments.

Dentifrices: Effects on supragingival calculus

References

Bánóczy, J., Sári, K., Schiff, T., Petrone, M., Davies, R. & Volpe, A.R. (1995) Anticalculus efficacy of three dentifrices. American Dental Journal 8, 205-208.

Fairbrother, K.J., Kowolik, M.J., Curzon, M.E.J., Müller, I., McKeown, S., Hill, C.M., Hannigan, C., Bartizek, R.D. & White, D.J. (1997) The comparative clinical efficacy of pyrophosphate/triclosan, copolymer/triclosan and zinc citrate/triclosan dentifrices for the reduction of supragingival calculus formation. Journal of Clinical Dentistry 8, 62-66.

Lobene, R.R. (1987) A clinical comparison of the anticalculus effect of two commercially-available dentifrices. Clinical Preventive Dentistry 9 (4), 3-8.

Schiff, T.G. (1987) The effect of a dentifrice containing soluble pyrophosphate and sodium fluoride on calculus deposits. A 6-month clinical study. Clinical Preventive Dentistry 9 (2), 13-16.

Volpe, A.R., Schiff, T.J., Cohen, S., Petrone, M.E. & Petrone, D. (1992) Clinical comparison of the anticalculus efficacy of two triclosan-containing dentifrices. Journal of Clinical Dentistry 3, 93-95.

White, D.J., McClanahan, S.F., Lanzalaco, A.C., Cox, E.R., Bacca, L., Perlich, M.A., Campbell, S.A., Schiff, T. & Stains, A. (1996) The comparative efficacy of two commercial tartar control dentifrices in preventing calculus development and facilitating easier dental cleaning. Journal of Clinical Dentistry 7, 58-64.

SECTION 12

Dentifrices: Effects on dentine hypersensitivity

Dentifrices are available on the market with claims of reducing dentine hyper-sensitivity. Agents marketed as desensitizing include:

- Strontium chloride (Sensodyne-SC).

- Strontium acetate (Macleans Sensitive).

- Potassium nitrate (Aquafresh Sensitive, Colgate Sensitive/Tartar Control, Denquel, Promise with Fluoride, Sensitivity Protection Crest, Sensodyne-F, USA).

- Potassium chloride (Sensodyne-F, United Kingdom).

Dentine hypersensitivity is believed to originate from external irritation of open dentinal tubules, e.g. from thermal changes, sweet or sour foods. Strontium salts are thought to work by formation of deposits occluding open dentinal tubules. Potassium salts are believed to have a desensitizing effect on pulpal nerve fibers. The desensitizing effects are commonly assessed by a combination of methods:

- *Tactile sensitivity examination:* The tip of an adjustable pressure sensitive probe is passed over the exposed cervical area. During examination, the probing force is increased step-wise in increments of 10 g from 10 g to 70 g. The force required to cause discomfort is used as a measure of the degree of sensitivity.

- *Cold air sensitivity examination:* The cervical area is exposed to a blast of air from a dental air syringe for 1 second using a standardized pressure and a temperature of about 70°F (20°C). The patient grades the pain by placing a mark on a 100 mm long line marked with "no pain" and "excruciating pain" at the ends. The distance in mm from the "no pain" end of the line to the mark is used as a measure of degree of sensitivity (Visual Analog Scale, VAS).

- *Subjective assessment:* The patient is asked to rate the overall degree of pain from the sensitive teeth in the dentition by placing a mark on a VAS.

Three recent trials representing the desensitizing agents above are selected for review in this section.

STUDIES PRESENTED IN THIS SECTION

Authors	Page	Subjects	Dentifrices	Observation interval
Silverman et al. (1996)	185	Adults with hyper-sensitive teeth	Strontium chloride Potassium nitrate Potassium nitrate/fluoride Placebo	8 weeks
Gillam et al. (1996)	188	Adults with hyper-sensitive teeth	Strontium acetate/fluoride Potassium chloride/fluoride Control fluoride	6 weeks
West et al. (1997)	191	Adults with hyper-sensitive teeth	Strontium acetate/fluoride Potassium nitrate/fluoride Control fluoride	6 weeks

SILVERMAN ET AL. (1996) compared the effects of a strontium chloride dentifrice, a potassium nitrate dentifrice, a potassium nitrate/fluoride dentifrice and a placebo dentifrice.

Subjects and procedures:

* 220 subjects, 19-77 years of age, with ≥1 teeth responding to both tactile and cold air stimuli at each of 2 repeated baseline examinations (interval not reported)

* 1-2 teeth per subject selected for test

* Study groups (parallel design):
    - Strontium chloride dentifrice: strontium chloride (10%) in diatomaceous earth abrasive base (Sensodyne-SC) (N=60)

    - Potassium nitrate dentifrice: potassium nitrate (5%) in ?[†] abrasive base (Denquel) (N=50)

    - Potassium nitrate/fluoride dentifrice: potassium nitrate (5%) + sodium fluoride (0.243%) in ?[†] abrasive base (Sensitivity Protection Crest) (N=50)

    - Placebo dentifrice: without strontium, potassium or fluoride in ?[†] abrasive base (N=60)

* Subjects received a soft toothbrush and the assigned toothpaste, were instructed to brush their teeth 2 x daily, and to cover the entire length of the brush head with dentifrice

* Dentine hypersensitivity measurements (see page 183):
    - tactile sensitivity examination (probing force, 10-70 g)
    - cold air sensitivity examination (VAS rating, 0-100 mm)
    - subjective assessment (VAS rating, 0-100 mm)

* 8 weeks of observation

* Analyses of mean results for tactile sensitivity, cold air sensitivity and subjective overall pain assessment

[†] Not mentioned by the authors.

Results:

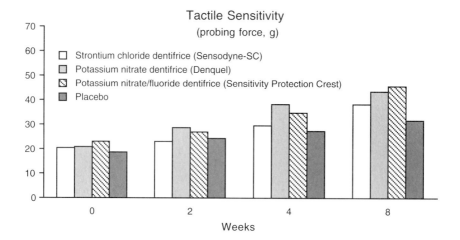

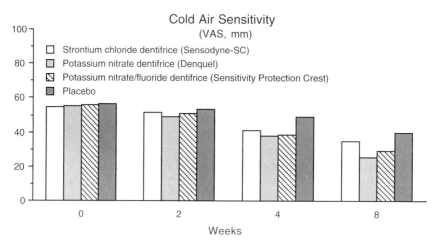

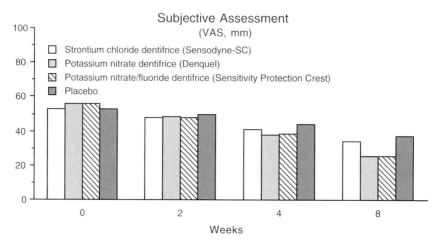

Comments:

- The degree of hypersensitivity gradually decreased for all 4 study groups during the 8-week observation interval as determined from all 3 methods of evaluation (tactile sensitivity, cold air sensitivity and subjective assessment by the patients).

- Reduced sensitivity was also observed for the placebo group (no active ingredient, no fluoride). This may hypothetically be explained as follows:
  - A placebo effect, commonly noticed in studies on drugs in general as well as studies on dentine hypersensitivity, related to psychological/physiological reactions caused by a desire by the patient to obtain relief of symptoms and possibly also to please the therapist.
  - Patients participating in a hypersensitivity study may improve the cleaning of the sensitive teeth. Reduced levels of plaque over the hypersensitive areas may allow for deposits of calcium salts from the saliva, occluding open dentinal tubules.
  - A natural and gradual improvement of hypersensitivity over time. Dentine hypersensitivity may 'spontaneously' decrease and increase in afflicted persons. Since the selection of subjects for study is based upon a minimum number of sensitive teeth or a minimum degree of sensitivity, a certain number of participant may have been selected on their peak of natural sensitivity variation. This would effect the overall results for each study group of subjects, resulting in an average decrease of sensitivity.

- Compared to the placebo group, decrease in sensitivity was enhanced for the 3 specially formulated toothpastes. The relative improvements following use of the strontium chloride dentifrice, however, were limited.

- The finding that the specially formulated dentifrices reduced hypersensitivity beyond that of a placebo dentifrice is in keeping with results of a multitude of studies published over the years (see reviews by Kanapka 1990 and Zappa 1994; and more recent studies by Nagata et al. 1994, Schiff et al. 1994 and Silverman et al. 1994).

- Addition of sodium fluoride to the potassium nitrate dentifrice for the sake of caries protection did not seem to reduce or enhance the desensitizing effect of the dentifrice. Likewise, addition of sodium monofluorophosphate to a potassium chloride dentifrice did not alter the desensitizing effect (Silverman et al. 1994).

GILLAM ET AL. (1996) compared the effects of a strontium acetate/fluoride dentifrice, a potassium chloride/fluoride dentifrice and a fluoride control dentifrice.

Subjects and procedures:

* 56 subjects, 18-60 years of age, with ≥2 teeth responding to both tactile and cold air stimuli

* Study groups (parallel design):
  - Strontium acetate/fluoride dentifrice: strontium acetate (8%) + sodium fluoride (0.23%) in silica abrasive base (Maclean's Sensitive) (N=19)

  - Potassium chloride/fluoride dentifrice: potassium chloride (3.75%) + sodium monofluorophosphate (0.8%) in calcium phosphate abrasive base (Sensodyne-F) (N=18)

  - Control fluoride dentifrice: sodium monofluorophosphate (0.75%) + calcium glycerophosphate (0.13%) + sodium fluoride (0.016%) in ?[†] abrasive base (Aquafresh) (N=19)

* Subjects received a toothbrush and the assigned toothpaste, and were instructed to brush their teeth at least for 1 minute 2 x daily

* Dentine hypersensitivity measurements:
  - tactile sensitivity examination (probing force, 10-70 g)
  - cold air sensitivity examination (VAS rating, 0-100 mm)
  - subjective assessment (VAS rating, 0-100 mm)

* 6 weeks of observation

* Analyses of mean results for tactile sensitivity, cold air sensitivity and subjective overall pain assessment

[†] Not mentioned by the authors.

Results:

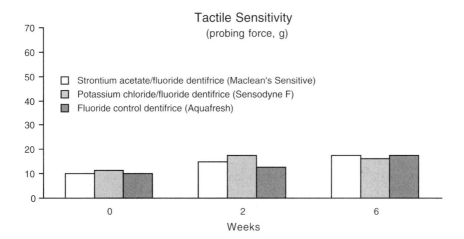

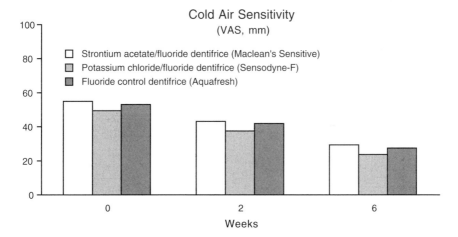

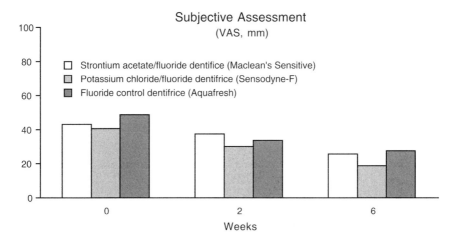

Comments:

- The degree of hypersensitivity decreased for all 3 study groups during the 6-week observation interval as determined from all 3 methods of evaluation (tactile sensitivity, cold air sensitivity and subjective assessment by the patients).

- The results of this study, thus, indicate that the decrease in sensitivity following use of a sodium fluoride/sodium monofluorophosphate dentifrice corresponds to the decreases for the specially formulated dentifrices.

- A 4th study group - placebo without active ingredients and without fluoride - would have been desirable. This would have indicated how much of the improvements that could be ascribed to the placebo effect.

WEST ET AL. (1997) compared the effects of a strontium acetate/fluoride dentifrice, a potassium nitrate/fluoride dentifrice and a control fluoride dentifrice.

Subjects and procedures:
* 112 subjects, 18-65 years of age, with ≥2 teeth responding to cold air stimulus at 2 repeated baseline examinations, 4 weeks apart during use of a fluoride toothpaste

* Study group (parallel design):
  - Strontium acetate/fluoride dentifrice: strontium acetate (8%) + sodium fluoride (0.23%) in silica abrasive base (Maclean's Sensitive) (N=38)

  - Potassium nitrate/fluoride dentifrice: potassium nitrate (?%[†]) + sodium fluoride (?%[†]) in ?[†] abrasive base (Aquafresh Sensitive) (N=37)

  - Control fluoride dentifrice: sodium monofluorophosphate (0.75%) + calcium glycerophosphate (0.13%) + sodium fluoride (0.016%) in ?[†] abrasive base (Aquafresh) (N=37)

* Subjects received a soft toothbrush and the assigned toothpaste, and were instructed to brush their teeth 2 x daily

* Dentine hypersensitivity measurements:
  - tactile sensitivity examination (VAS rating following manual probing, 0-10)
  - cold air sensitivity examination (VAS rating, 0-10)
  - subjective assessment (VAS rating, 0-10)

* 6 weeks of observation

* Analyses of mean results for tactile sensitivity, cold air sensitivity and subjective overall pain assessment

[†] Not mentioned by the authors.

Results:

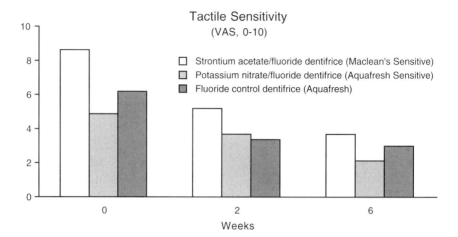

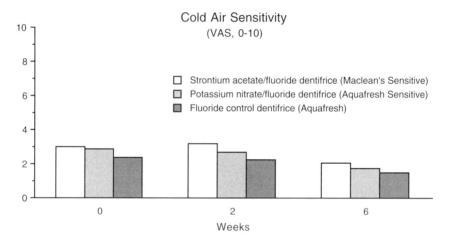

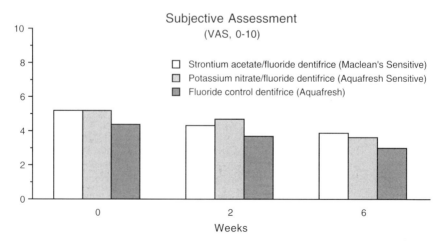

Comments:

- The degree of hypersensitivity decreased for all 3 study groups during the 6-week observation interval as determined from all 3 methods of evaluation (tactile sensitivity, cold air sensitivity and subjective assessment by the patients).

- Similar to the results of Gillam et al. (1996) (pages 188-190), the findings of this study indicate that the decrease in sensitivity following use of a sodium fluoride/sodium monofluorophosphate dentifrice (Aquafresh) corresponds to the decreases for the specially formulated dentifrices. In a previous study by the same research group, another sodium fluoride/sodium monofluoro-phosphate dentifrice (Colgate) produced corresponding decrease in sensitivity as a strontium chloride dentifrice (Sensodyne-SC) and a strontium ace-tate/fluoride dentifrice (Maclean's Sensitive) (Pearce et al. 1994).

- A 4th study group - placebo without active ingredients and without fluoride - would have been desirable. This would have indicated the degree of improvement that could be ascribed to the placebo effect.

Dentifrices: Effects on dentine hypersensitivity

Concluding remarks

Dentifrices with strontium chloride, strontium acetate, potassium nitrate or potassium chloride may provide alleviation of dentine hypersensitivity beyond that of an inactive placebo following treatment periods over 6-8 weeks.

Sodium fluoride/sodium monofluorophosphate dentifrices have been observed to provide similar degree of desensitization as specially formulated dentifrices in 3 recent studies.

The majority of dentifrices on the market contain fluoride. This may justify the choice of a fluoride dentifrice for control rather than the use of a placebo (without active ingredient and without fluoride). Specially formulated dentifrices may only be warranted if they provide effects superior to those of regular fluoride dentifrices. Ideally, future studies should include both a placebo and a fluoride control dentifrice to allow evaluation of the placebo effect as well as a comparison to a regular fluoride dentifrice. (The use of the term placebo dentifrice may not be entirely correct in this context, since it can not be excluded that the other dentifrice ingredients may have some effects on dentine hypersensitivity.)

Since strontium salts and potassium salts are supposed to alleviate dentine hypersensitivity through different mechanisms, it can not be excluded that some patients may respond better to the one salt than the other. This reasoning may also apply to fluoride dentifrices. It appears that our approaches to treatment are troubled by our lack of knowledge of the etiology of dentine hypersensitivity.

Few studies have investigated the duration of the sensitivity decrease following cessation of use of a desensitizing dentifrice. Addy et al. (1987) found slight indications of sensitivity return 6 weeks following a previous 6-week use of each of 2 strontium acetate dentifrices. Gillam et al. (1992) also found a limited recurrence of sensitivity 12 weeks following a previous 8-week use of each of 2 strontium chloride dentifrices. It would be valuable if follow-ups were included as an integral part of future trials.

Dentifrices: Effects on dentine hypersensitivity

References

Addy, M., Mostafa, P. & Newcombe, R. (1987) Dentine hypersensitivity: a comparison of five toothpastes used during 6-week treatment period. British Dental Journal 163, 45-51.

Gillam, D.G., Newman, H.N., Bulman, J.S. & Davies, E.H. (1992) Dentifrice abrasivity and cervical dentinal hypersensitivity. Results 12 weeks following cessation of 8 weeks' supervised use. Journal of Periodontology 63, 7-12.

Gillam, D.G., Bulman, J.S., Jackson, R.J. & Newman, H.N. (1996) Comparison of 2 desensitizing dentifrices with a commercially available fluoride dentifrice in alleviating cervical dentine sensitivity. Journal of Periodontology 67, 737-742.

Kanapka, J.A. (1990) Over-the-counter dentifrices in the treatment of tooth hypersensitivity. Dental Clinics of North America 34 (3), 545-560.

Nagata, T., Ishida, H., Shinohara, H., Nishikawa, S., Kasahara, S., Wakano, Y., Daigen, S. & Troullos, E.S. (1994) Clinical evaluation of a potassium nitrate dentifrice for the treatment of dentinal hypersensitivity. Journal of Clinical Periodontology 21, 217-221.

Pearce, N.X., Addy, M. & Newcombe R.G. (1994) Dentine hypersensitivity: A clinical trial to compare 2 strontium desensitizing toothpastes with a conventional fluoride toothpaste. Journal of Periodontology 56, 113-119.

Schiff, T., Dotson, M., Cohen, S., DeVizio, W., McCool, J. & Volpe, A. (1994) Efficacy of a dentifrice containing potassium nitrate, soluble pyrophosphate, PVM/MA copolymer, and sodium fluoride on dentinal hypersensitivity: A twelve-week clinical study. Journal of Clinical Dentistry 5 (spec. issue), 87-92.

Silverman, G., Gingold, J. & Curro, F.A. (1994) Desensitizing effect of a potassium chloride dentifrice. American Dental Journal 7, 9-12.

Silverman, S., Berman, E., Hanna, C.B., Salvato, A., Fratarcangelo, P., Bartizek, A.D., Bollmer, B.W., Campbell, S.L., Lanzalaco, A.C., Mackay, B.J., McClanahan, S.F., Perlich, M.A. & Shaffer, J.B. (1996) Assessing the efficacy of three dentifrices in the treatment of dentinal hypersensitivity. Journal of American Dental Association 127, 191-201.

West, N.X., Addy, M., Jackson, R.J. & Ridge, D.B. (1997) Dentine hypersensitivity and the placebo response. A comparison of the effect of strontium acetate, potassium nitrate and fluoride toothpastes. Journal of Clinical Periodontology 24, 209-215.

Zappa, U. (1994) Self-applied treatment in the management of dentine hypersensitivity. Archives of Oral Biology 39 (suppl.), 107S-112S.

Mouthrinses: Effects on plaque and gingivitis

As yet, there are no mouthrinses available which are effective enough and without side effects to allow for long-term substitution of mechanical plaque control methods. With the products at hand, the focus needs to be limited to the following questions:

- Are there any agents that are effective enough and without significant side effects during short-term periods of use when mechanical plaque control methods are unsuited, e.g. postoperatively after oral surgical procedures?

- Are there any agents that can provide adjunctive effects, without side effects, during long-term use as a supplement to mechanical plaque control?

Among available antimicrobial mouthrinse compounds are:
- Amine fluoride/stannous fluoride (Meridol)
- Cetylpyridinium chloride (e.g. Cepacol)
- Cetylpyridinium chloride/domiphen bromide (e.g. Scope)
- Chlorhexidine (Corsodyl, Peridex)
- Oxygenating agents (Perimed)
- Phenolic essential oils (Listerine)
- Sanguinarine (Viadent)
- Sanguinarine/zinc chloride (PerioGard Veadent, Viadent)
- Triclosan/copolymer (Actibrush, Colgate Plax, Colgate Total)

The literature does not include sufficient research for a comprehensive evaluation and comparison of different mouthrinses. In this section, 2 studies on short-term substitution of mechanical plaque control are selected for review. Effects of long-term use of mouthrinses to supplement mechanical plaque control are illustrated by results of 3 trials.

Sanguinarine/zinc chloride mouthrinses have primarily been evaluated following combined use with sanguinarine/zinc chloride containing dentifrices. An example of results from such combined use is also included.

STUDIES PRESENTED IN THIS SECTION

Authors	Page	Subjects	Agents	Alone/ Supplement	Observation interval
Siegrist et al. (1986)	199	Dental students/ assistants	Chlorhexidine, 0.12% Phenolic essential oils Sanguinarine Placebo	Alone	21 days
Brecx et al. (1990)	202	Nondental students	Chlorhexidine, 0.20% Phenolic essential oils Amine fluoride/ stannous fluoride Placebo	Alone	21 days
Segreto et al. (1986)	205	Adults	Chlorhexidine, 0.12% Chlorhexidine, 0.20% Placebo	Supplement	3 months
Grossman et al. (1989)	209	Adults with some evidence of gingivitis	Phenolic essential oils Chlorhexidine, 0.12% Sanguinarine Placebo	Supplement	6 months
Worthington et al. (1993)	213	Adults with plaque and gingivitis	Triclosan/copolymer Placebo	Supplement	6 months
Kopczyk et al. (1991)	216	Adults with plaque and gingivitis	Sanguinarine/zinc chloride mouthrinse + dentifrice Placebo	Supplement	6 months

SIEGRIST ET AL. (1986) compared the plaque and gingivitis inhibiting effects of mouthrinses with chlorhexidine, phenolic essential oils and sanguinarine as the only oral hygiene measure during 3 weeks.

Subjects and procedures:
* 31 dental students and assistants, 19-28 years of age

* 4 study groups (parallel design, 'experimental gingivitis' model):
    - Chlorhexidine gluconate, 0.12% (N=9)
    - Phenolic essential oils (Listerine) (N=9)
    - Sanguinarine (Viadent) (N=9)
    - Placebo (flavored alcoholic solution) (N=4)

* 2-week pretreatment phase with initial prophylaxis and instructions in optimal mechanical plaque control to achieve healthy baseline gingival conditions

* Following baseline examination, subjects were asked to refrain from mechanical plaque control

* Mouthrinses 2 x daily (mornings and evenings) with assigned rinse according to manufacturers instructions; supervised during week-days, unsupervised during week-ends

* Plaque scores at 4 locations of each tooth using Silness-Löe index (scores 0-3)

* Gingivitis scores at 4 locations of each tooth using Löe-Silness index (scores 0-3)

* Extrinsic tooth stain assessed from photographs of buccal and lingual surfaces of all teeth using Lang-Räber discoloration index (scores 0-3; 0 = none; 1 = slight; 2 = moderate; 3 = heavy)

* 21 days of observation

* Analyses of mean plaque, gingivitis and stain index scores

Results:

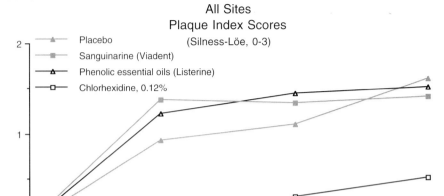

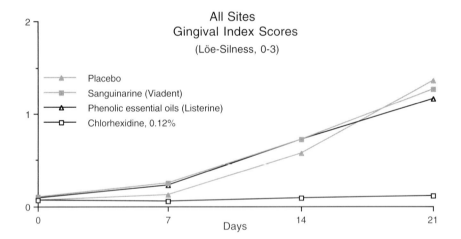

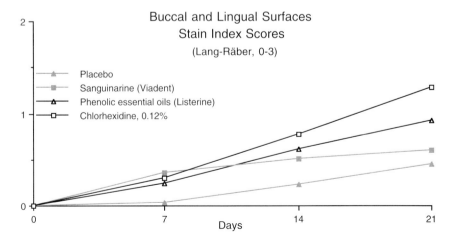

Comments:

- Compared to the other treatment groups, accumulation of dental plaque and development of gingivitis were markedly retarded for the 0.12% chlorhexidine group.

- The plaque index scores for the Listerine and Viadent groups levelled off after increases during the initial 7 days. This may in part be explained by the plaque index used, which evaluates plaque at the gingival margin only. A plaque index system scoring the extension of plaque over the tooth surfaces may have shown a different result.

- Small numbers of subjects were included in the experimental groups, particularly in the placebo group. It is well known from 'experimental gingivitis' studies that individual subjects accumulate plaque and develop gingivitis at various rates. It can not be excluded that the groups may have had different proportions of slow and rapid plaque/gingivitis formers. This may have affected the results. The lower plaque scores for the placebo group at 7 and 14 days compared to Listerine and Viadent groups is probably an effect of such an imbalance.

- More extrinsic tooth stain tended to accumulate following use of chlorhexidine than following the other agents. This finding is supported by similar observations in other 'experimental gingivitis' studies (Moran et al. 1988, 1991).

BRECX ET AL. (1990) compared the plaque and gingivitis inhibiting effects of mouthrinses with chlorhexidine, phenolic essential oils and an amine fluoride/stannous fluoride compound as the only oral hygiene measure during 3 weeks.

Subjects and procedures:
* 36 nondental students, 20-34 years of age

* 4 study groups (parallel design, 'experimental gingivitis' model):
    - Chlorhexidine gluconate, 0.20% (N=9)
    - Phenolic essential oils (Listerine) (N=9)
    - Amine fluoride/stannous fluoride compound (Meridol) (N=10)
    - Placebo (0.02% quinine-hydrochloride solution) (N=8)

* 2-week pretreatment phase with initial prophylaxis and instructions in optimal mechanical plaque control to achieve healthy baseline gingival conditions

* Following baseline examination, subjects were asked to refrain from mechanical plaque control, and to use assigned rinse 2 x daily, 10 ml for 1 minute

* Plaque scores at 4 locations of each tooth using Silness-Löe index (scores 0-3)

* Gingivitis scores at 4 locations of each tooth using Löe-Silness index (scores 0-3)

* 21 days of observation

* Analyses of mean plaque and gingivitis scores

Results:

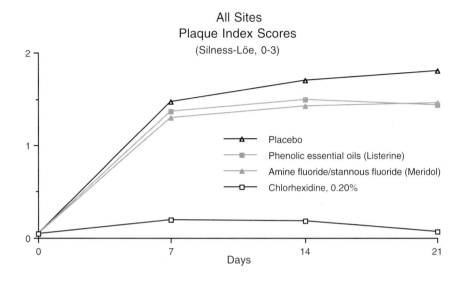

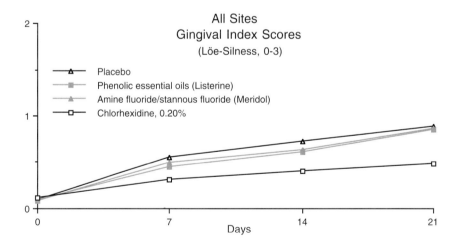

Comments:

- Compared to the other treatment groups, accumulation of dental plaque was markedly retarded for the 0.20% chlorhexidine group. Overall, results for plaque formation of this study compare well to those of Siegrist et al. (1986) (pages 199-201).

- Less gingivitis developed for 0.20% chlorhexidine group than for the other groups. Compared to Siegrist et al. (1986) (pages 199-201) the difference in favor of chlorhexidine was more limited. Again, the low number of subjects in these studies may be part of the explanation. The difference in gingivitis results may also be related to different interpretations/applications of the gingival index scoring system.

- Extrinsic tooth stain was not recorded.

- Although results of the 2 studies reviewed above on use of mouthrinses alone vary somewhat, results of other 'experimental gingivitis' studies confirm that rinses with 0.12% or 0.20% chlorhexidine are superior to other agents available and tested so far (Moran et al. 1988, 1991, Quirynen et al. 1990).

- There seems to be no 'experimental gingivitis' study where 0.12% chlorhexidine and 0.20% chlorhexidine have been directly compared.

SEGRETO ET AL. (1986) evaluated the effects of daily mouthrinses with 0.12% and 0.20% chlorhexidine to supplement mechanical tooth cleaning.

Subjects and procedures:

* Originally 597 adults with gingivitis, but without advanced periodontitis

* Study groups, matched for age, sex and gingivitis (parallel design):
    - Chlorhexidine gluconate, 0.12% (original N=199)
    - Chlorhexidine gluconate, 0.20% (original N=202)
    - Placebo (without chlorhexidine) (original N=196)

* Following baseline examination, all subjects received prophylaxis (plaque score = 0), a soft toothbrush and a standard toothpaste, were instructed to continue their normal mechanical tooth cleaning, and to use provided mouthrinse 2 x daily, 15 ml during 30 seconds

* Plaque scores at 6 locations of each tooth using disclosing dye and Turesky/ Quigley-Hein index (scores 0-5)

* Gingivitis scores at 6 locations of each tooth using Löe-Silness index (scores 0-3)

* 12 weeks of observation

* Analyses of mean plaque and gingivitis scores and % gingivitis-free sites

Results:

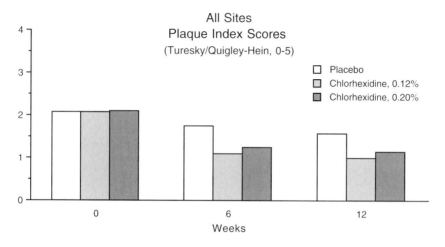

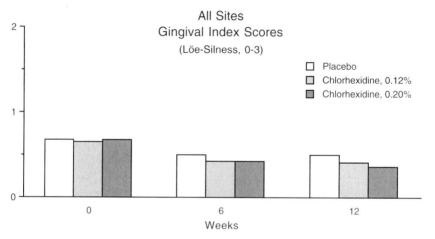

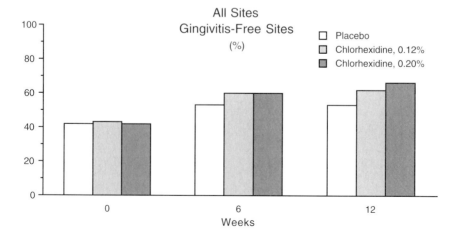

Comments:

- Plaque scores for the placebo group were lower at 6 and 12 weeks than at baseline prior to prophylaxis. The scores for 0.12% and 0.20% chlorhexidine groups were additionally reduced, and to a similar degree for both groups.

- The gingivitis scores for the placebo group were also lower at 6 and 12 weeks than at baseline. The reduction could be related to the prophylaxis provided at baseline and to a participation effect.

- Gingivitis levels for 0.12% and 0.20% chlorhexidine groups at 6 and 12 weeks were somewhat lower than those for the placebo, both expressed as mean gingivitis scores and % gingivitis-free sites in the dentition. The scores were similar for both chlorhexidine groups.

- Comparison of results for anterior and posterior parts of the dentition, and for buccal, lingual and proximal sites would have been of interest.

- 20% of all participants did not complete 6 weeks of study, and 26% of subjects did not complete 12 weeks of study. For their analyses of baseline and 6-week data, the authors opted to include subjects that had discontinued at a later stage, since they found that balance between groups for baseline scores of plaque and gingivitis was maintained also following loss of subjects.

- It was stated that there were no findings "which would indicate that adverse effects were produced by either chlorhexidine mouthrinse in comparison to the placebo mouthrinse".

- Recordings of extrinsic tooth stain accumulation were not performed.

- The results of this trial are supported by findings of Axelsson & Lindhe (1987), evaluating 2 x daily supervised mouthrinses during 60 seconds with 0.10% chlorhexidine and 0.20% chlorhexidine as a supplement to mechanical tooth cleaning over 6 weeks in adults. Compared to placebo, use of both concentrations of chlorhexidine resulted in similarly and significantly improved plaque and gingivitis scores. In this study, however, 8 of 24 individuals in the 0.20% group developed oral mucosal lesions (unspecified), but none in the 0.10% group.

- In studies on chlorhexidine, accumulation of typical tooth and tongue stain enables the examiners to identify participants of chlorhexidine groups, which means that they lose their examiner 'blindness'. Grossman et al. (1986) encountered this problem by covering the teeth with custom made opaque plastic onlays and the tongue with a paste of food colors. Final 6-month recordings by 2 different examiners in their study showed similar scores with and without the use of tooth and tongue covers for both examiners. Any corresponding type of precaution was not taken in the study reviewed above by Segreto et al. (1986).

GROSSMAN ET AL. (1989) compared the effects of daily mouthrinses with chlorhexidine, phenolic essential oils and sanguinarine to supplement mechanical tooth cleaning.

Subjects and procedures:
* 502 adults with ≥1 sites with bleeding on probing, but without signs of overt periodontitis

* Study groups, matched for age and gingivitis (parallel design):
    - Chlorhexidine gluconate, 0.12% (Peridex) (N=113)
    - Phenolic essential oils (Listerine) (N=129)
    - Sanguinarine (Viadent) (N=127)
    - Placebo ('Peridex' without chlorhexidine) (N=133)

* Following baseline examination, subjects received a soft toothbrush and a standard toothpaste, were instructed to continue their normal mechanical tooth cleaning, and to use provided mouthrinse 2 x daily as directed by manufacturer

* No baseline prophylaxis

* Plaque scores at facial and lingual aspects of each tooth using disclosing dye and Turesky/Quigley-Hein index (scores 0-5)

* Gingivitis scores at 6 locations of each tooth using Löe-Silness index (scores 0-3)

* Extrinsic dental stain assessed from photographs of buccal surfaces of maxillary and mandibular anterior teeth; composite index of stain intensity (scores 0-4) and stain area (scores 0-6)

* 6 months of observation

* Analyses of mean plaque, gingivitis and stain index scores

Results:

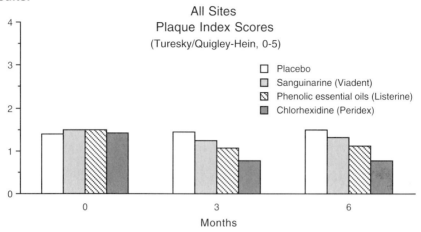

All Sites
Plaque Index Scores
(Turesky/Quigley-Hein, 0-5)

☐ Placebo
▨ Sanguinarine (Viadent)
▨ Phenolic essential oils (Listerine)
▨ Chlorhexidine (Peridex)

Months

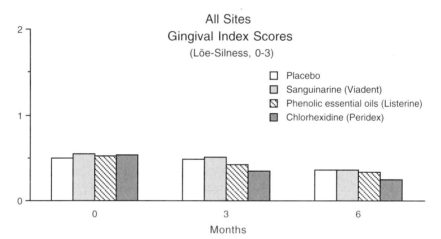

All Sites
Gingival Index Scores
(Löe-Silness, 0-3)

☐ Placebo
▨ Sanguinarine (Viadent)
▨ Phenolic essential oils (Listerine)
▨ Chlorhexidine (Peridex)

Months

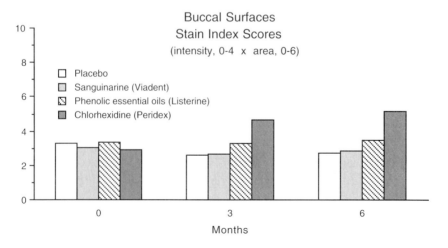

Buccal Surfaces
Stain Index Scores
(intensity, 0-4 x area, 0-6)

☐ Placebo
▨ Sanguinarine (Viadent)
▨ Phenolic essential oils (Listerine)
▨ Chlorhexidine (Peridex)

Months

Comments:

- Baseline plaque scores were relatively low. Compared to baseline and the placebo group, plaque scores at 3 and 6 months were slightly reduced in the Viadent group, more noticeably in the Listerine groups and markedly in the Peridex group.

- Baseline gingivitis scores were also comparatively low. Compared to placebo, scores were lower at 3 and 6 months for the Peridex group. Overall, gingivitis scores were lower at 6 months than at 3 months. Result of examiner drift?

- Gingivitis was graded a 2nd time at 6 months using masking devices for the teeth and the tongue. Similar overall scores were obtained with and without the use of these devices (data not shown here).

- Comparison of results for anterior and posterior parts of the dentition, and for buccal, lingual and proximal sites would have been of interest.

- Use of Peridex resulted in increased stain index scores. Accumulation of extrinsic tooth stain following use of Peridex to supplement mechanical tooth cleaning but not following use of Listerine was also observed by Overholser et al. (1990) in a 6-month study.

- It was stated that "examinations of the oral mucosa were conducted to detect pathoses which could possibly be attributed to product use". Results of these examinations, however, were not given. Nevertheless, other studies have examined the oral mucosa following use of 0.12% chlorhexidine and Listerine over 6-9 months and found no indication of soft tissue effects (Gordon et al. 1985, Grossman et al. 1986, DePaola et al. 1989, Overholser et al. 1990).

- Other trials on mouthrinses with 0.12% chlorhexidine as a supplement to mechanical tooth cleaning have also found similar degrees of reductions of plaque and bleeding scores compared to placebo (Grossman et al. 1986, 6 months of observation; Segreto et al. 1986, 3 months of observation, pages 205-208; Banting et al. 1989, 2 years of observation; Eaton et al. 1997, 3 months of observation).

- Other studies on Listerine to supplement mechanical tooth cleaning support the findings that use of this agent may reduce plaque and bleeding scores somewhat compared to placebo (Lamster et al. 1983, 6 months of observation; Gordon et al. 1985, 9 months of observation; DePaola et al. 1989, 6 months of observation; Overholser et al. 1990; 6 months of observation).

WORTHINGTON ET AL. (1993) studied the effects of a pre-brush mouthrinse with triclosan/copolymer.

Subjects and procedures:

* 117 adults, 18-65 years of age, with plaque and gingivitis, but no probing depths ≥5 mm

* Study groups (parallel design):
    - Triclosan/copolymer (Colgate Plax) (N=60)
    - Placebo (without triclosan/copolymer) (N=57)

* Following baseline examination, subjects received the assigned mouthrinse, a soft toothbrush and a standard toothpaste, were instructed to rinse mornings and evenings for 60 seconds with 15 ml of assigned rinse, and to brush their teeth for 30 seconds immediately thereafter

* No baseline prophylaxis

* Plaque scores of 'overnight plaque' at 6 locations of each tooth using disclosing dye and Turesky/Quigley-Hein index (scores 0-5)

* Gingivitis scores at 6 locations of each tooth using Löe-Silness index (scores 0-3)

* 6 months of observation

* Analyses of mean plaque and gingivitis scores

Results:

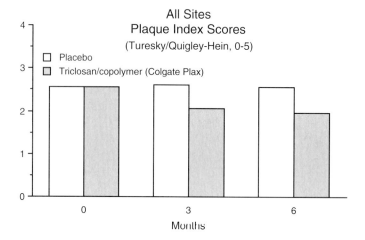

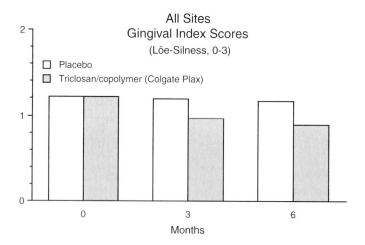

Comments:

- Compared to baseline and placebo group, plaque and gingivitis scores were reduced in the Colgate Plax group at 3 and 6 months.

- Comparison of results for anterior and posterior parts of the dentition, and for buccal, lingual and proximal sites would have been of interest.

- The authors did not offer any explanation for the choice of 30 seconds of toothbrushing only.

- The authors stated that "no side effects were observed or reported throughout the study".

- In similar 6-month studies on the same pre-brush rinse, corresponding reductions of plaque and gingivitis scores have been obtained (Ayad & Berta 1995, Triratana et al. 1995). Absence of soft tissue and extrinsic stain side effects were also reported in these studies.

- Colgate Plax has also been marketed under the names of Actibrush (Colgate) and Colgate Total. This triclosan/copolymer agent is different from Plax (Phizer) or Advanced Formula Plax (Phizer), containing detergents as 'active' ingredients. Plax (Phizer) has been extensively evaluated and found ineffective in almost all of studies (e.g. Lobene et al. 1990, 6 months of observation; O'Mullane et al. 1994, 12 months of observation). Advanced Formula Plax (Phizer), although less investigated, may also have questionable effectiveness (Schiff & Borden 1994, 6 months of observation; Cronin et al. 1997, 6 weeks of observation).

KOPCZYK ET AL. (1991) studied the effects of combined use of dentifrices and mouthrinses containing sanguinarine/zinc chloride to supplement mechanical plaque control.

Subjects and procedures:

* 113 adults ≥18 years (mean ages 26-27 years) with Turesky/Quigley-Hein plaque index score ≥2 and bleeding on probing score ≥50%, but without signs of periodontitis

* Study groups (parallel design):
  - Sanguinarine/zinc chloride dentifrice in dicalcium phosphate base (Viadent original, nonfluoride) + sanguinarine/zinc chloride mouthrinse (Viadent) (Active, nonfluoride group; N=27)
  - Placebo nonfluoride dentifrice + placebo mouthrinse (Placebo, nonfluoride group; N=30)
  - Sanguinarine/zinc chloride/fluoride dentifrice in silica base (Viadent fluoride) + sanguinarine/zinc chloride mouthrinse (Viadent) (Active, fluoride group; N=27)
  - Placebo fluoride dentifrice + placebo mouthrinse (Placebo, fluoride group; N=29)

* Following baseline examination, subjects received a soft toothbrush and the assigned dentifrice + mouthrinse, were instructed to continue their normal brushing and flossing 2 x daily for 1 minute followed by use of 15 ml of provided mouthrinse for 1 minute, and to refrain from drinking, eating, rinsing or smoking for 30 minutes after use of products

* No baseline prophylaxis

* Reinforcement by supervised brushing + rinsing following recordings at each visit for examination

* Plaque scores at facial and lingual aspects of each tooth using disclosing dye and Turesky/Quigley-Hein index (scores 0-5)

* Gingivitis scores for buccal and lingual papillae and gingival margins of all teeth using Lobene index (scores 0-4)

* Bleeding on probing scores (% of examined sites); site locations not given

* 6 months of observation

* Analyses of mean plaque, gingivitis and bleeding on probing scores

Results:

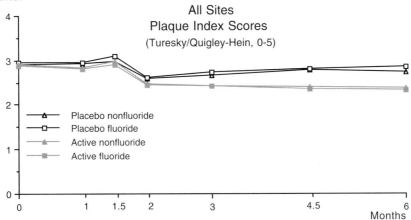

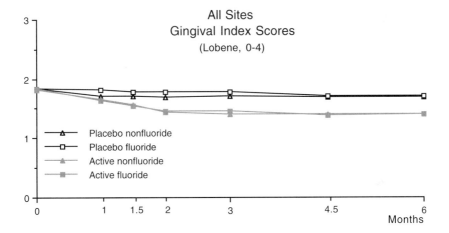

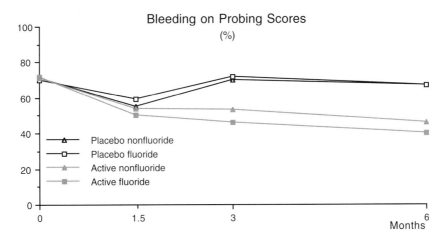

Comments:

- Improved results were observed for both active groups as compared to both placebo groups for plaque index scores, gingival index scores as well as bleeding on probing scores.

- Comparison of results for anterior and posterior parts of the dentition, and for buccal, lingual and proximal sites would have been of interest.

- The relative benefits of the sanguinarine/zinc chloride mouthrinse versus sanguinarine/zinc chloride dentifrice can not be determined from this study, and do not seem to have been investigated.

- It was reported that 2 subjects of the active nonfluoride group showed some mucosal irritation, possibly related to the products used.

- Microbial samples obtained from the buccal mucosa and the dorsum of the tongue for evaluation of yeast and Gram-negative bacilli did not disclose any opportunistic overgrowths (data not shown here). Extended microbiological analyses in another 6-month study also did not reveal any opportunistic overgrowths (Harper et al. 1990b).

- The antiplaque and antigingivitis effects of the combined use of sanguinarine/zinc chloride mouthrinse and sanguinarine/zinc chloride dentifrice are supported by results of a 6-month study by Harper et al. (1990a).

- Cullinan et al. (1997) studied the combined use of sanguinarine/zinc chloride dentifrice and mouthrinse to supplement personal plaque control during 4-6 visits of active nonsurgical periodontal treatment and 6 weeks of subsequent follow-up. Improvements of plaque scores, gingivitis scores and probing depths were similar for sanguinarine/zinc chloride and placebo groups.

Mouthrinses: Effects on plaque and gingivitis

Concluding remarks

Mouthrinses with 0.12% or 0.20% chlorhexidine seem to be an effective oral hygiene measure during short-term periods when mechanical plaque control is unsuitable, e.g. postoperatively after oral surgical procedures. Extrinsic tooth stain, however, will accumulate.

Mouthrinses with chlorhexidine (Corsodyl, Peridex), triclosan/copolymer (Acti-brush, Colgate Plax, Colgate Total) and maybe also phenolic essential oils (Listerine) may have some adjunctive plaque inhibiting effects as supplements to mechanical plaque control. The effects on gingivitis, however, seem more limited and may have questionable clinical significance. This includes chlorhexidine, which unfortunately results in accumulation of extrinsic tooth stain, also when used together with toothbrushing with a standard dentifrice.

Mouthrinses with cetylpyridinium chloride (e.g. Cepacol) as supplement to mechanical plaque control have been evaluated in 6-week studies. The results have been equivocal and do not allow any conclusions on efficacy (Ashley et al. 1984, Finkelstein et al. 1990, Moran & Addy 1991, Nelson et al. 1991).

There appears to be no longer-term study published on the effects of mouthrinses with cetylpyridinium chloride/domiphen bromide (e.g. Scope).

The oxygenating mouthrinse Perimed has been evaluated when combined with professional subgingival irrigation every 3rd week (Clark et al. 1989), but seemingly not following use of mouthrinse alone to supplement mechanical plaque control.

Mouthrinses with sanguinarine (Viadent - without zinc chloride) seem to have little or no adjunctive effect as supplement to mechanical plaque control.

Sanguinarine/zinc chloride mouthrinses (PerioGard Veadent, Viadent) do not seem to have been tested in longer-term trials. However, studies on the combined use of sanguinarine/zinc chloride mouthrinses and sanguinarine/zinc chloride dentifrices suggest that this combined use may have some antiplaque and antigingivitis effects as supplements to mechanical plaque control, although this was not confirmed in a 6-week follow-up of initial periodontal therapy.

Short-term studies on mouthrinses have demonstrated that the effects on plaque and gingivitis vary within the dentition. Increased efficacy has been observed for buccal aspects as compared to lingual aspects of the teeth, and for incisors as compared to molars (e.g. Axelsson & Lindhe 1987, Ramberg et al. 1992). It would have been advantageous if the available longer-term mouthrinse trials had presented results for various tooth groups and site locations. Again, data on % plaque-free and % gingivitis-free proximal sites would seem to the most relevant way of assessing the efficacy of mouthrinses to supplement mechanical plaque control.

Mouthrinses: Effects on plaque and gingivitis

References

Ashley, F.P., Skinner, A., Jackson, P., Woods, A. & Wilson, R.F. (1984) The effect of a 0.1% cetylpyridinium chloride mouthrinse on plaque and gingivitis in adult subjects. British Dental Journal 157, 191-196.

Axelsson, P. & Lindhe, J. (1987) Efficacy of mouthrinses in inhibiting dental plaque and gingivitis in man. Journal of Clinical Periodontology 14, 205-212.

Ayad, F. & Berta, R. (1995) Effect on plaque removal and gingivitis of a triclosan-copolymer pre-brush rinse: A six-month clinical study in Canada. Journal of Canadian Dental Association 61, 53-61.

Banting, D., Bosma, M. & Bollmer, B. (1989) Clinical effectiveness of a 0.12% chlorhexidine mouthrinse over two years. Journal of Dental Research 68, spec. issue, 1716-1718.

Brecx, M., Netuschil, L., Reichert, B. & Schreil, G. (1990) Efficacy of Listerine, Meridol and chlorhexidine mouthrinses on plaque, gingivitis and plaque bacteria vitality. Journal of Clinical Periodontology 17, 292-297.

Clark, W.B., Magnusson, I., Walker, C.B. & Marks, R.G. (1989) Efficacy of Perimed® antibacterial system on established gingivitis. (I). Clinical results. Journal of Clinical Periodontology 16, 630-635.

Cronin, M., Gordon, J. & Fernandez, P. (1997) Two independent clinical trials comparing pre-brush mouthrinse formulations in reducing supragingival plaque. Journal of Canadian Dental Association 63, 347-355.

Cullinan, M.P., Powell, R.N., Faddy, M.J. & Seymour, G.J. (1997) Efficacy of a dentifrice and oral rinse containing sanguinaria extract in conjunction with initial periodontal therapy. Australian Dental Journal 42, 47-51.

DePaola, L.G., Overhholser, C.D., Meiller, T.F., Minah, G.E. & Niehaus, C. (1989) Chemotherapeutic inhibition of supragingival dental plaque and gingivitis development. Journal of Clinical Periodontology 16, 311-315.

Eaton, K.A., Rimini, F.M., Zak, E., Brookman, D.J., Hopkins, L.M.A., Cannell, P.J., Yates, L.G., Morrice, C.A., Lall, B.A. & Newman H.N. (1997) The effects of a 0.12% chlorhexidine-digluconate-containing mouthrinse versus a placebo on plaque and gingival inflammation over a 3-month period. A multicentre study carried out in general dental practices. Journal of Clinical Periodontology 24, 189-197.

Finkelstein, P., Yost, K.G. & Grossman, E. (1990) Mechanical devices versus antimicrobial rinses in plaque and gingivitis reduction. Clinical Preventive Dentistry 12, (3), 8-11.

Gordon, J.M., Lamster, I.B. & Seiger, M.C. (1985) Efficacy of Listerine antiseptic in inhibiting the development of plaque and gingivitis. Journal of Clinical Periodontology 12, 697-704.

Grossman, E., Reiter, G., Sturzenberger, O.P., de la Rosa, M., Dickinson, T.D., Ferretti, G.A., Ludlam, G.E. & Meckel, A.H. (1986) Six-month study of the effects of a chlorhexidine mouthrinse on gingivitis in adults. Journal of Periodontal Research, suppl., 33-43.

Grossman, E., Meckel, A.H., Isaacs, R.L., Ferretti, G.A., Sturzenberger, O.P., Bollmer, B.W., Moore, D.J., Lijana, R.C. & Manhart, M.D. (1989) A clinical comparison of antibacterial mouthrinses: Effects of chlorhexidine, phenolics, and sanguinarine on dental plaque and gingivitis. Journal of Periodontology 60, 435-440.

Harper, D.S., Mueller, L.J., Fine, J.B., Gordon, J. & Laster, L.L. (1990a) Clinical efficacy of a dentifrice and oral rinse containing sanguinaria extract and zinc chloride during 6 months of use. Journal of Periodontology 61, 352-358.

Harper, D.S., Mueller, L.J., Fine, J.B., Gordon, J. & Laster, L.L. (1990b) Effect of 6 months use of and dentifrice and oral rinse containing sanguinaria extract and zinc chloride upon the microflora of the dental plaque and oral soft tissues. Journal of Periodontology 61, 359-363.

Kopczyk, R.A., Abrams, H., Brown, A.T., Matheny, J.L. & Kaplan, A.L. (1991) Clinical and microbiological effects of a sanguinaria-containing mouthrinse and dentifrice with and without fluoride during 6 months of use. Journal of Periodontology 62, 617-622.

Lamster, I.B., Alfano, M.C., Seiger, M.C. & Gordon, J.M. (1983) The effect of Listerine antiseptic on reduction of existing plaque and gingivitis. Clinical Preventive Dentistry 5, (6), 12-16.

Lobene, R.R., Soparkar, P.M. & Newman, M.B. (1990) Long-term evaluation of a prebrushing dental rinse for the control of dental plaque and gingivitis. Clinical Preventive Dentistry 12, (2), 26-30.

Moran, J. & Addy, M. (1991) The effects of a cetylpyridinium chloride prebrushing rinse as an adjunct to oral hygiene and gingival health. Journal of Periodontology 62, 562-564.

Moran, J., Addy, M. & Newcombe, R. (1988) A clinical trial to assess the efficacy of sanguinarine-zinc mouthrinse (Veadent) compared with chlorhexidine mouthrinse (Corsodyl). Journal of Clinical Periodontology 15, 612-616.

Moran, J., Pal, D., Newcombe, R. & Addy, M. (1991) Comparison of a phenolic and a 0.2% chlorhexidine mouthrinse on the development of plaque and gingivitis. Clinical Preventive Dentistry 13, (4), 31-35.

Nelson, R.F., Rodasti, P.C., Tichnor, A. & Lio, Y.L. (1991) Comparative study of four over-the-counter mouthrinses claiming antiplaque and/or antigingivitis benefits. Clinical Preventive Dentistry 13, (6), 30-33.

O´Mullane, D.M., Whelton, H., Galvin, N., Phelan, J. & Gleeson, P. (1994) A 12-month study of the efficacy of a pre-brushing rinse in plaque removal. Journal of Periodontology 65, 611-615.

Overholser, C.D., Meiller, T.F., DePaola, L.G., Minah, G.E. & Niehaus, C. (1990) Comparative effects of 2 chemotherapeutic mouthrinses on the development of supragingival dental plaque and gingivitis. Journal of Clinical Periodontology 17, 575-579.

Quirynen, M., Marechal, M. & van Steenberghe, D. (1990) Comparative antiplaque activity of sanguinarine and chlorhexidine in man. Journal of Clinical Periodontology 17, 223-227.

Ramberg, P., Furuichi, Y., Lindhe, J. & Gaffar, A. (1992) A model for studying the effects of mouthrinses on de novo plaque formation. Journal of Clinical Periodontology 19, 509-520.

Schiff, T. & Borden, L.C. (1994) The effect of a new experimental prebrushing dental rinse on plaque removal. Journal of Clinical Dentistry 4, 107-110.

Segreto, V.A., Collins, E.M., Beiswanger, B.B., de la Rosa, M., Isaacs, R.L., Lang, N.P., Mallatt, M.E. & Meckel, A.H. (1986) A comparison of mouthrinses containing two concentrations of chlorhexidine. Journal of Periodontal Research, suppl., 23-32.

Siegrist, B.E., Gusberti, F.A., Brecx, M.C., Weber, H.P. & Lang, N.P. (1986) Efficacy of rinsing with chlorhexidine gluconate in comparison to phenolic and plant alkaloid compounds. Journal of Periodontal Research, suppl., 60-73.

Triratana, T., Kraivaphan, P., Amornchat, C., Rostogi, K., Petrone, M. & Volpe, A.R. (1995) Effect of a triclosan/copolymer pre-brush mouthrinse on established plaque formation and gingivitis: A six-month clinical study in Thailand. Journal of Clinical Dentistry 6, 142-147.

Worthington, H.V., Davies, R.M., Blinkhorn, A.S., Mankodi, S., Petrone, M., DeVizio, W. & Volpe, A.R. (1993) A six-month clinical study on the effect of a pre-brush rinse on plaque removal and gingivitis. British Dental Journal 175, 322-326.

SECTION 14

Mouthrinses: Effects on oral malodor

Bad breath (halitosis) commonly originates from the oral cavity. Volatile sulphide gases like hydrogen sulphide and methyl mercaptan, produced by microbial putrefaction of proteins, give rise to malodor. The microbial aggregations in untreated periodontal disease may produce malodor. In individuals with healthy periodontal conditions, bacterial accumulations on the dorsum of the tongue may be a source of bad breath.

Antimicrobial, breath freshening mouthrinses are available on the market. Only 10 studies, however, seem to have been published on the effects of mouthrinses on oral malodor. Five of these studies are reviewed here.

The deodorizing effects have been assessed by a combination of 2 methods:

- *Organoleptic measurement:* The odorous quality of exhaled mouth air is assessed by an odor judge, placed behind a screen to maintain judge and donor anonymity. The subject exhales mouth air into a tube passing through the screen. The judge rates the degree of malodor following sniffing the exhaled air, using a scale which may extend from 0 (no appreciable odor) to 5 (extremely foul odor). Mean scores from 2 or more independent judges have also been used.

- *Volatile sulphides measurements:* The concentration of volatile sulphides in samples of mouth air is measured using gas chromatography, or more recently using portable sulphide monitors developed for the purpose of oral malodor assessments.

STUDIES PRESENTED IN THIS SECTION

Authors	Page	Subjects	Mouthrinses	Observation interval
Schmidt & Tarbet (1978)	227	Adults with oral malodor	Zinc chloride mouthrinse Saline No treatment	3 hours
Pitts et al. (1983)	230	Adults with oral malodor	Phenolic essential oils Placebo Water	3 hours
Rosenberg et al. (1992)	233	Dental students	Chlorhexidine, 0.20% 2 phase oil/water mouthrinse Placebo	24 hours
Bosy et al. (1994)	236	Adults with oral malodor	Chlorhexidine, 0.20% + tongue brushing	1 week
Kozlovsky et al. (1996)	238	University students	Phenolic essential oils 2 phase oil/water mouthrinse	6 months

SCHMIDT & TARBET (1978) studied the effect of a zinc chloride mouthrinse on oral malodor over 3 hours.

Subjects and procedures:

* 62 adult volunteers with no obvious oral pathology and with baseline organoleptic malodor score ≥1 (see below)

* Study groups (parallel design):
    - Zinc chloride mouthrinse (Lavoris) (N=21)

    - Saline mouthrinse (N=21)

    - No treatment (N=20)

* Subjects abstained from eating, drinking and oral hygiene on the day of test until completion of recordings

* Organoleptic assessment of the mouth air by a panel of 3 independent judges using a scale from 0 to 3 (0 = no malodor, 1 = low to moderate; 2 = moderate to high; 3 = high malodor)

* Measurements of concentrations of hydrogen sulphide and methyl mercaptan in samples of mouth air using gas chromatography

* 3 hours of observation

* Analyses of mean results for organoleptic scores and concentrations of hydrogen sulphide and methyl mercaptan

Results:

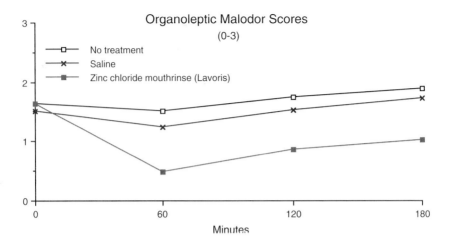

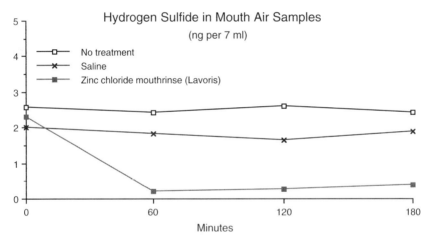

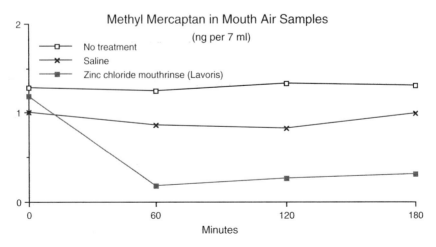

Comments:

- Reduced levels of malodor were observed during 3 hours following rinses with the zinc chloride mouthrinse (Lavoris) as observed from the organoleptic scores, although a gradual return towards baseline values could be observed (means of scores from 3 independent judges).

- Concentrations of the volatile odorous substances hydrogen sulphide and methyl mercaptan remained reduced during the entire 3-hour period following rinses with Lavoris.

- Data for continued measurements beyond 3 hours would have been of interest.

PITTS ET AL. (1983) studied the effect of a phenolic essential oils mouthrinse on oral malodor over 3 hours.

Subjects and procedures:

* 30 adult volunteers with no obvious oral pathology and with baseline concentrations of methyl mercaptan of ≥30 parts per billion in samples of mouth air

* Study groups (cross-over design):
    - Phenolic essential oils mouthrinse (Listerine)

    - Placebo mouthrinse (without phenolic essential oils)

    - Water mouthrinse

* Subjects reported to the laboratory 7:00-8:00 a.m. on test days having abstained from eating, drinking and oral hygiene since arising, and from smoking for 1 hour; also having abstained from eating garlic and onion-containing foods on the evening prior to the test day

* Supervised rinsing with 20 ml of assigned mouthrinse during 30 seconds; "in random order on different test days"

* Organoleptic assessment of the mouth air by a panel of 5 independent judges using a scale from 1 to 9 (1 = extremely pleasant; 5 = neutral; 9 = extremely unpleasant)

* Measurements of concentrations of hydrogen sulphide and methyl mercaptan in samples of mouth air using gas chromatography

* 3 hours of observation

* Analyses of mean results for organoleptic scores and concentrations of hydrogen sulphide and methyl mercaptan

Results:

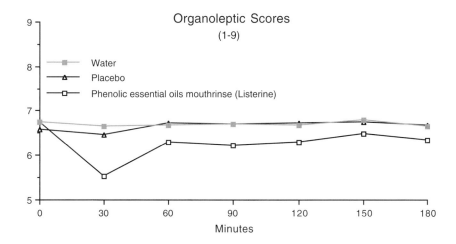

Organoleptic Scores (1-9)

Water
Placebo
Phenolic essential oils mouthrinse (Listerine)

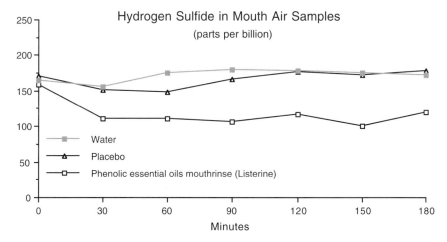

Hydrogen Sulfide in Mouth Air Samples (parts per billion)

Water
Placebo
Phenolic essential oils mouthrinse (Listerine)

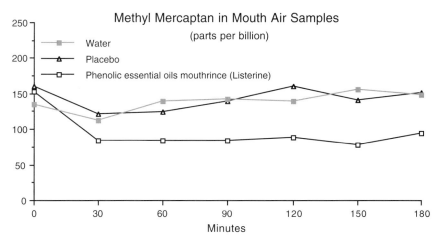

Methyl Mercaptan in Mouth Air Samples (parts per billion)

Water
Placebo
Phenolic essential oils mouthrince (Listerine)

Comments:

- Reduced levels of malodor were observed during 3 hours following rinses with the phenolic essential oils mouthrinse (Listerine) as observed from the organoleptic scores (means of scores from 5 independent judges). The 'clinical significance' of the mean difference compared to placebo and water rinses is somewhat difficult to appreciate - a difference of about 0.5 unit on a scale from 5 (neutral) to 9 (extremely unpleasant).

- Concentrations of the volatile odorous substances hydrogen sulphide and methyl mercaptan were also lower following rinses with Listerine as compared to placebo and water.

- The drop of the organoleptic scores after 30 minutes was not paralleled by corresponding reductions of the levels of volatile sulphide gases at this time point. This may be an indication of the masking effect of the mouthwash flavors on the malodor.

- Data for continued measurements beyond 3 hours would have been of interest.

- This study seems to be a follow-up of a previous publication by the same research group using a similar design, but limited to 2 hours of observation. In this previous study, Listerine was also found to reduce the organoleptic scores to some extent compared to rinses with water (Pitts et al. 1981). Somewhat surprisingly, there seem to be no additional studies published by this research group to follow-up on these short-term findings.

ROSENBERG ET AL. (1992) studied the effects of a chlorhexidine mouthrinse and a 2 phase oil/water mouthrinse on oral malodor over 24 hours.

Subjects and procedures:

* 60 dental students

* Study groups (parallel design):
    - Chlorhexidine, 0.20% mouthrinse (Corsodyl) (N=19)

    - 2 phase oil/water mouthrinse: aqueous phase with 0.05% cetylpyridinium chloride; oil phase with olive oil and phenolic essential oils (Agis, Israel) (N=22)

    - Placebo mouthrinse (N=19)

* Baseline measurements between 4:00-6:00 p.m. on day 1

* Instructions to rinse with assigned mouthrinse during 30 seconds at bedtime on day 1 and after arising on day 2, and to refrain from rinsing with water, eating or drinking for 30 minutes after rinses

* Final measurements between 4:00-6:00 p.m. on day 2

* Organoleptic assessment of the mouth air by a single judge, using a scale from 0 to 5 (0 = no appreciable odor; 5 = extremely foul odor)

* Measurements of concentrations of volatile sulphides in samples of mouth air using a sulphide monitor

* 24 hours of observation

* Analyses of mean results for organoleptic scores and concentrations of volatile sulphides

Results:

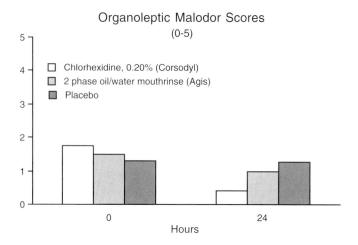

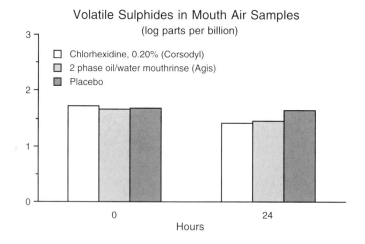

Comments:

- Rinses with chlorhexidine at bedtime and in the morning reduced the organoleptic malodor scores of afternoon mouth air. The effect on volatile sulphide levels was less noticeable, although statistically significant as compared to placebo.

- For the 2 phase oil/water mouthrinse, only the reduction of volatile sulphide levels reached statistical significance.

- Dental students were included as subjects in this study irrespective of their baseline scores. A corresponding study limited to subjects with pre-experimental objectional malodor would have been of interest.

BOSY ET AL. (1994) studied the effects of the combination of daily chlorhexidine mouthrinse and tongue brushing on oral malodor over 7 days.

Subjects and procedures:

* 101 patients reporting oral malodor and attending a Halitosis Assessment
  Clinic

* Baseline recordings followed by 2 consecutive study periods of each 1 week:
  - Week 1: No treatment
  - Week 2: 2 x daily tongue brushing with a toothbrush soaked in 0.20%
    chlorhexidine + 60-sec mouthrinse with 0.20% chlorhexidine

* Subjects asked to refrain from rinsing with water for 30 minutes after rinses

* Subjects requested to abstain from eating, drinking, chewing, brushing and
  mouthrinsing for 2 hours prior to each recording

* Organoleptic assessment of the mouth air by a single judge, using a scale
  from 0 to 5 (0 = no odor; 5 = extremely foul odor)

* Measurements of concentrations of volatile sulphides in samples of mouth air
  using a sulphide monitor

* Analyses of mean results for organoleptic scores and concentrations of
  volatile sulphides

Results:

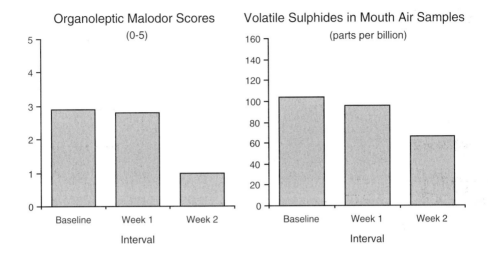

Comments:

- The combination of tongue brushing and rinses with chlorhexidine caused a reduction of both organoleptic malodor scores and volatile sulphide levels.

- The results of this study are supported by findings of De Boever & Loesche (1995) using the same consecutive-week design.

- The relative contributions of tongue brushing and use of chlorhexidine can not be determined from any of these 2 studies. (For effects of tongue brushing alone on oral malodor, see pages 133-134.)

KOZLOVSKY ET AL. (1996) studied the effects of a phenolic essential oils mouthrinse and a 2 phase oil/water mouthrinse on oral malodor over 6 months.

Subjects and procedures:
* 50 nonsmoking university students

* Study groups (parallel design):
    - Phenolic essential oils mouthrinse (Listerine) (N= 24)

    - 2 phase oil/water mouthrinse: aqueous phase with 0.05% cetylpyridinium chloride; oil phase with olive oil and phenolic essential oils (Assuta, Israel) (N= 26)

* Instructions to rinse mornings and evenings with assigned mouthrinse for 30 seconds, and to refrain from rinsing with water, eating or drinking for 30 minutes after rinses

* Organoleptic assessment of the mouth air by 2 independent judges, using a scale from 0 to 5 (0 = no appreciable odor; 5 = extremely foul odor)

* Measurements of concentrations of volatile sulphides in samples of mouth air using a sulphide monitor

* Gingivitis scores for buccal and lingual papillae and gingival margins of 6 representative teeth in the dentition ('Ramfjord teeth') using Lobene index (scores 0-4)

* 6 months of observation

* Analyses of mean results for organoleptic scores, concentrations of volatile sulphides and gingival index

Results:

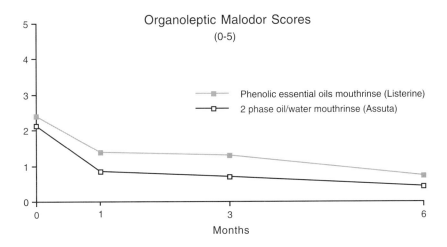

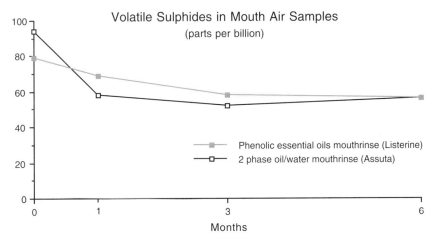

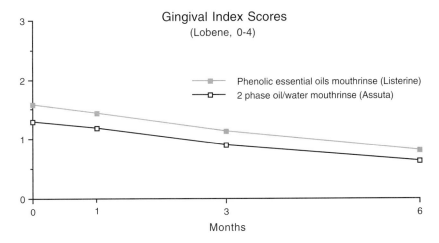

Comments:

- The results of this study are difficult to interpret due to the imbalance of baseline scores for mouth air and gingivitis measurements, and due to lack of control group. The recorded improvements of the malodor measurements could possibly be related to improved mechanical plaque control due to a participation effect.

- The gradual decrease of the gingivitis scores would tend to support the possibility of a participation effect.

- This appears to be the only long-term study available on effects of mouthrinses on oral malodor.

Mouthrinses: Effects on oral malodor

Concluding remarks

Mouthrinses with antimicrobial agents containing phenolic essential oils (Listerine) and zinc chloride (Lavoris) seem to have some effects on malodor during periods of 2-3 hours. Effects following mouthrinses with chlorhexidine (Corsodyl, Peridex) may possibly be of longer duration, although this has not been sufficiently investigated.

For pilot studies on mouthrinses, it may be practical to include subjects without any requirement of a minimum level of malodor. However, it appears that final and more relevant investigation should be performed in individuals with more objectionable mouth odor as determined from repeated pre-experimental measurements.

The limited number of studies available on mouthrinses and oral malodor is surprising in view of the abundant commercial supply of various agents. Additional studies are highly needed.

No study on effects of oral sprays on oral malodor has been identified. In one study, chewing gum, breath mints and oxidizing lozenges were investigated. Effects on oral malodor seemed inconclusive (Bar-Ness Greenstein et al. 1997).

Mouthrinses: Effects on oral malodor

References

Bar-Ness Greenstein, R., Goldberg, S., Marku-Cohen, S., Sterer, N. & Rosenberg, M. (1997) Reduction of oral malodor by oxidizing lozenges. Journal of Periodontology 68, 1176-1181.

Bosy, A., Kulkatni, G.V., Rosenberg, M. & McCulloch, C.A.G. (1994) Relationship of oral malodor to periodontitis: Evidence of independence in discrete subpopulations. Journal of Periodontology 65, 37-46.

De Boever, E.H. & Loesche, W.J. (1995) Assessing the contribution of anaerobic microflora of the tongue to oral malodor. Journal of the American Dental Association 126, 1384-1393.

Kozlovsky, A., Goldberg, S., Natour, I., Rogatky-Gat, A., Gelernter, I. & Rosenberg, M. (1996) Efficacy of a 2 phase oil:water mouthrinse in controlling oral malodor, gingivitis and plaque. Journal of Periodontology 67, 577-582.

Pitts, G., Pianotti, R., Feary, T.W., McGuiness, J. & Masurat, T. (1981) The in vivo effect of an antiseptic mouthwash on odor-producing microorganisms. Journal of Dental Research 60, 1891-1896.

Pitts, G., Brogdon, C., Hu, L., Masurat, T., Pianotti, R. & Schumann, P. (1983) Mechanism of action of an antiseptic, anti-odor mouthwash. Journal of Dental Research 62, 738-742.

Rosenberg, M., Gelernter, I., Barki, M. & Bar-Ness, R. (1992) Day-long reduction of oral malodor by a two phase oil:water mouthrinse as compared to chlorhexidine and placebo rinses. Journal of Periodontology 63, 39-43.

Schmidt, N.F. & Tarbet, W.J. (1978) The effect of oral rinses on organoleptic mouth odor ratings and levels of volatile sulfur compounds. Oral Surgery, Oral Medicine & Oral Pathology 45, 876-883.

Dental irrigation

Pulsating irrigation devices for the purpose of self-applied supragingival irrigation of the teeth have intermittently been promoted over the years, starting from
the 1960's. Initially, use of water irrigation for plaque and gingivitis control was
investigated. Later, irrigation with antimicrobial agents has also been evaluated.

Chlorhexidine has been found more effective than other antimicrobial mouth
rinsing agents (See Section 13: Mouthrinses: Effects on Plaque and Gingivitis,
pages 197-223). This section includes reviews of 2 studies comparing the effects
over 6 months of chlorhexidine mouthrinse, irrigation with water and irrigation
with chlorhexidine to supplement mechanical plaque control.

STUDIES PRESENTED IN THIS SECTION

Authors	Page	Subjects	Agent/ Delivery	Observation interval
Flemmig et al. (1990)	245	Adults with gingivitis	Chlorhexidine, 0.12% rinse Chlorhexidine, 0.06% irrigation Water irrigation Control	6 months
Chaves et al. (1994)	248	Adults with gingivitis	Chlorhexidine, 0.12% rinse Chlorhexidine, 0.04% irrigation Water irrigation Control	6 months

FLEMMIG ET AL. (1990) compared the effects of mouthrinses with chlorhexidine, irrigation with chlorhexidine and irrigation with water to supplement mechanical plaque control.

Subjects and procedures:
* 175 adults with ≥6 sites with bleeding on probing, but no probing depth ≥5 mm (details on any attachment loss/interdental papillary heights not provided)

* Study groups, matched for sex and gingivitis:
  - Chlorhexidine, 0.12% rinse (Peridex): 15 ml 2 x daily for 30 seconds (N=43)
  - Chlorhexidine, 0.06% irrigation (Peridex diluted 1:2): pulsating irrigation 1 x daily (evenings) with 300 ml water followed by 200 ml chlorhexidine using WaterPik (N=40)
  - Water irrigation: pulsating irrigation 1 x daily (evenings) with 500 ml water using WaterPik (N=44)
  - Control: mechanical plaque control alone (N=48)

* Following baseline examination, subjects received prophylaxis, instructions in WaterPik use (irrigation groups), asked to continue their normal mechanical tooth cleaning and to use the provided toothbrush and toothpaste

* Plaque scores at 6 locations of each tooth using Silness-Löe index (scores 0-3)

* Bleeding on probing scores at 6 locations of each tooth (presence/absence, % of examined sites)

* Extrinsic dental stain assessed from photographs of buccal surfaces of maxillary and mandibular anterior teeth (composite intensity/area stain index, details not explained)

* 6 months of observation

* Analyses of mean plaque, bleeding on probing and stain scores

Results:

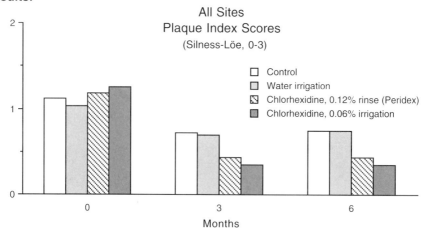

All Sites
Plaque Index Scores
(Silness-Löe, 0-3)

☐ Control
▨ Water irrigation
▨ Chlorhexidine, 0.12% rinse (Peridex)
■ Chlorhexidine, 0.06% irrigation

Months

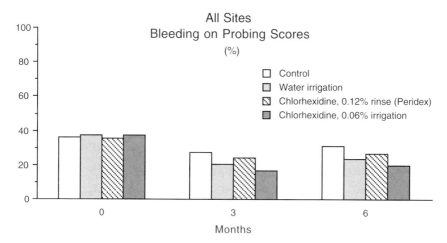

All Sites
Bleeding on Probing Scores
(%)

☐ Control
▨ Water irrigation
▨ Chlorhexidine, 0.12% rinse (Peridex)
■ Chlorhexidine, 0.06% irrigation

Months

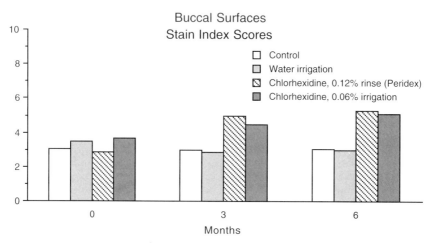

Buccal Surfaces
Stain Index Scores

☐ Control
▨ Water irrigation
▨ Chlorhexidine, 0.12% rinse (Peridex)
■ Chlorhexidine, 0.06% irrigation

Months

Comments:

- Compared to control group, plaque scores at 3 and 6 months were reduced in the chlorhexidine rinse and chlorhexidine irrigation groups, but not in the water irrigation group.

- Compared to control group, bleeding on probing scores at 3 and 6 months were slightly reduced in the water irrigation and the chlorhexidine rinse groups and somewhat more noticeably in the chlorhexidine irrigation group.

- Participation effects were apparent in this study as observed from the results of the control group.

- Use of chlorhexidine rinse and chlorhexidine irrigation resulted in increased stain index scores.

- Chlorhexidine rinse and chlorhexidine irrigation also resulted in increased formation of supragingival calculus on the lingual aspects of the mandibular anterior teeth (data not presented here). Increased calculus formation following use of chlorhexidine has also been reported by others (e.g. Overholser et al. 1990).

- The authors reported that 1 patient in the chlorhexidine irrigation group was excluded due to development of epithelial desquamation of the ventral surface of the tongue. No other soft tissue side effects were mentioned.

CHAVES ET AL. (1994) also compared the effects of mouthrinses with chlorhexidine, irrigation with chlorhexidine and irrigation with water to supplement mechanical plaque control.

Subjects and procedures:
* 104 adults, 19-62 years of age, with bleeding on probing score ≥30%, and ≤4 sites with probing depth ≥7 mm (details on any attachment loss/interdental papillary heights not provided)

* Study groups:
    - Chlorhexidine, 0.12% rinse (Peridex): 15 ml 2 x daily for 30 seconds (N=24)
    - Chlorhexidine, 0.04% irrigation (Peridex diluted 1:3): irrigation 1 x daily with 400 ml using WaterPik (N=21)
    - Water irrigation: irrigation 1 x daily with 400 ml water using WaterPik (N=32)
    - Control: mechanical plaque control alone (N=27)

* Following baseline examination, subjects received prophylaxis, video instruction in brushing and flossing, instruction in WaterPik use (irrigation groups), and asked to use the provided toothbrush and toothpaste

* Plaque scores at 6 locations of each tooth using Silness-Löe index (scores 0-3)

* Bleeding on probing scores at 6 locations of each tooth (presence/absence, % of examined sites)

* 6 months of observation

* Analyses of mean plaque and bleeding on probing scores

Results:

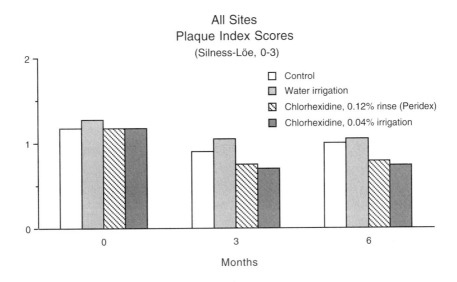

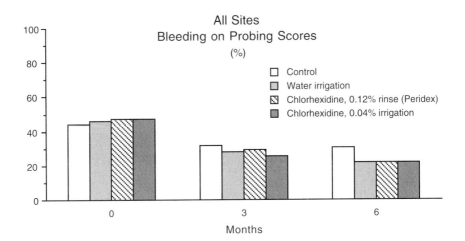

Comments:

- Compared to control group, plaque scores at 3 and 6 months were reduced in the chlorhexidine rinse and chlorhexidine irrigation groups, but not in the water irrigation group.

- Compared to control group, bleeding on probing scores at 6 months were somewhat reduced in the water irrigation group, in the chlorhexidine rinse group, and in the chlorhexidine irrigation group.

- Accumulations of stain and supragingival calculus were not recorded.

- The authors stated that "no patient reported adverse reaction or side effects to the mouthrinse or the irrigation device".

- The findings of this study are in accord with those of Flemmig et al. (1990) (pages 245-247). In both of these studies it was observed that water irrigation did not reduce plaque formation but showed some effect on gingivitis. This findings has also been made in several other studies (e.g. Newman et al. 1994, 6 months of observation).

- The results of both studies reviewed above indicate that there is little advantage to chlorhexidine irrigation (after dilution) over chlorhexidine mouthrinses, used as supplements to mechanical tooth cleaning.

- Irrigation with Listerine was compared to irrigation with a placebo solution in a 6-week study by Ciancio et al. (1989). Listerine, but not placebo irrigation, affected plaque scores somewhat. Gingivitis scores were slightly reduced by both irrigations.

Dental irrigation

Concluding remarks

Dental irrigation with water using available pulsating irrigation devices seems to provide some adjunctive gingivitis reducing effects when used to supplement mechanical plaque control. This effect has been observed without concomitant effects on recordings of plaque, including the use of an index focusing on the amounts of plaque along the gingival margin (Silness-Löe). The mechanism of the antigingivitis effects of water irrigation has not been clarified (Newman et al. 1990).

Irrigations with antimicrobials tested so far seem to provide little or no advantage over mouthrinses with these agents for the purpose of supplementing mechanical plaque control.

There seem to be no reports on the extent of continued use of irrigation devices following their recommendation.

Dental irrigation

References

Chaves, E.S., Kornman, K.S., Manwell, M.A., Jones, A.A., Newbold, D.A. & Wood, R.C. (1994) Mechanism of irrigation effects on gingivitis. Journal of Periodontology 65, 1016-1021.

Ciancio, S.G., Mather, M.L., Zambon, J.J. & Reynolds, H.S. (1989) Effect of a chemotherapeutic agent delivered by an oral irrigation device on plaque, gingivitis and subgingival microflora. Journal of Periodontology 60, 310-315.

Flemmig, T.F., Newman, M.G., Doherty, F.M., Grossman, E., Meckel, A.H. & Bakdash, M.B. (1990) Supragingival irrigation with 0.06% chlorhexidine in naturally occurring gingivitis. I. 6 month clinical observations. Journal of Periodontology 61, 112-117.

Newman, M.G., Flemmig, T.F., Nachnani, S., Rodrigues, A., Calsina, G., Lee, Y-S., de Camargo, P., Doherty, F.M. & Bakdash, M.B. (1990) Supragingival irrigation with 0.06% chlorhexidine in naturally occurring gingivitis. I. 6 month microbiological observations. Journal of Periodontology 61, 427-433.

Newman, M.G., Cattabriga, M., Etienne, D., Flemmig, T., Sanz, M., Kornman, K.S., Doherty, F., Moore, D.J. & Ross, C. (1994) Effectiveness of adjunctive irrigation in early periodontitis: Multi-center evaluation. Journal of Periodontology 65, 224-229.

Overholser, C.D., Meiller, T.F., DePaola, L.G., Minah, G.E. & Niehaus, C. (1990) Comparative effects of 2 chemotherapeutic mouthrinses on the development of supragingival dental plaque and gingivitis. Journal of Clinical Periodontology 17, 575-579.

SECTION 16

Oral hygiene instruction

In previous sections of this text, the efficacy of different oral hygiene methods have been evaluated in various groups of individuals. Limited differences have generally been observed between the tested methods. In addition, the overall impact on plaque and gingivitis scores during the course of the studies has usually been modest.

The limited overall impact could be explained by the fact that the participating subjects have typically been given no or little plaque control instruction at the start of the trials. This has been intentional, since investigators primarily have been interested in the efficacy of the oral hygiene methods under 'field' conditions, i.e. how the methods would work in the 'average' person without the provision of laborious instruction.

The present section focuses on what can be accomplished when the goal has been to reach maximum effectiveness of the oral hygiene instruction. More extensive instruction has been provided. Different modes of instruction have been compared in the search for cost-effective but yet adequate methods.

Six studies in adults representing these efforts are selected for review, each of them having at least 6 months of observation.

STUDIES PRESENTED IN THIS SECTION

SÖDERHOLM ET AL. (1982) compared the effectiveness of a 5-visit oral hygiene instruction program to that of a 2-visit program.

Subjects and procedures:

* 69 white-collar employees at a Swedish shipyard, 29-44 years of age

* 3 study groups matched for initial plaque scores and 5 other variables:
    - 5-visit group (N=23)
    - 2-visit group (N=23)
    - Control group (N=23)

* Initial examination (IN) followed by supragingival debridement of the teeth

* Baseline examination (B) and start of oral hygiene instruction (Visit I) at appointment 2 months later

* Oral hygiene instruction (personal, one-to-one)
    - 5-visit group: Step-by-step approach using 5 30-min appointments spaced 2-3 days apart during a 14-day period. Techniques and devices introduced gradually to allow the patients to realize the needs; use of plaque-disclosing dyes and illuminated mouth mirrors; feedback at each visit by charting tooth surfaces with plaque and calculation of plaque scores (% sites with plaque)
    - 2-visit group: 2 60-min visits spaced 7-10 days apart. Compared to the 5-visit program, more limited step-by-step approach and patient self-realization
    - Control group: Examinations only, no feedback. Instruction delayed until after the 6-week examination

* Recordings of presence/absence of plaque and bleeding on probing at 4 sites of each tooth (mesio-buccal, mid-buccal, disto-buccal and lingual)

* Short term follow-up after 2, 6 and 12 weeks

* All 3 groups provided periodontal and restorative treatment (Tx) after the 12-week examination

* Long-term follow-up during 4 years using recalls every 3rd month with oral hygiene reinforcement and supra- and subgingival debridement

* Analyses of mean plaque and bleeding scores (% sites with plaque/bleeding)

Results:

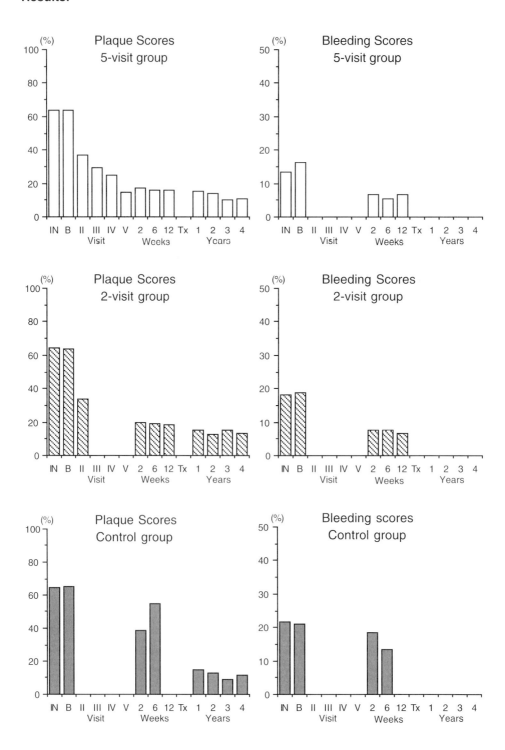

Comments:

- Initial supragingival debridement was performed in order to facilitate the subsequent plaque control for the patients. Baseline examination was delayed until 2 months later in order to ensure that any reduction in bleeding tendency resulting from this treatment would have occurred prior to the start of the experimental plaque control treatments.

- Similar short-term improvements of plaque and bleeding scores were observed for the 5-visit and 2-visit groups. These results indicate that the step-by-step teaching method included in the 5-visit program was not critical for short-term effectiveness of instruction.

- Initial bleeding on probing scores for the 3 study groups averaged 15-20 %. These comparatively low bleeding scores suggest that the subjects generally had limited periodontal involvement.

- The oral hygiene instructions were given by 2 dental assistants, each treating half the number of individuals in each experimental group. Separate analyses did not reveal any significant differences in effectiveness between the 2 assistants (data not shown here).

- The authors reported that analyses were also performed to study the effects separately for incisors + canines and for premolars + molars. Again, no differences were observed between the 5-visit and 2-visit programs.

- Some reductions of plaque and bleeding scores were also noted for the control group, demonstrating a participation effect.

- Plaque scores continued to remain low throughout the 4 years of observation in these white-collar workers provided frequent maintenance treatment. The long-term observations do not elucidate the long-term effects of the plaque control programs *per se* since the patients were given reinstruction as needed during maintenance.

SÖDERHOLM & EGELBERG (1982) used a 3-visit instruction program and compared the effectiveness of 30-min and 15-min appointments.

Subjects and procedures:

* 59 blue-collar employees at a Swedish shipyard, 38-47 years of age

* 3 study groups matched for initial plaque scores and 4 other variables:
    - 30-min group (N=20)
    - 15-min group (N=19)
    - Control group (N=20)

* Initial examination (IN) followed by supragingival debridement of the teeth

* Baseline examination (B) and start of oral hygiene instruction (Visit I) at appointment 4 months later

* Oral hygiene instruction (personal, one-to-one)
    30-min group:
      - Visit I: Complete instruction; use of plaque-disclosing dyes and illuminated mouth mirrors; charting of tooth surfaces with plaque and calculation of plaque scores (% sites with plaque)
      - Visit II & III (within 14 days): Feedback by charting tooth surfaces with plaque and calculation of plaque scores; renewed instruction at individual needs
    15-min group:
      - Visit I: As for the 30-min group but in a condensed form during 15 min
      - Visit II & III (within 14 days): Feedback by charting tooth surfaces with plaque and calculation of plaque scores; *no* renewed instructions
    Control group:
      - Examinations only, no feedback. Instruction delayed until after the 12-week examination

* Recordings of presence/absence of plaque at 4 sites of each tooth (mesio-buccal, mid-buccal, disto-buccal and lingual)

* Short term follow-up after 2, 6 and 12 weeks

* All 3 groups provided periodontal and restorative treatment (Tx) after the 12-week examination

* Long-term follow-up during 2 years using recalls every 3rd month with oral hygiene reinforcement and supra- and subgingival debridement

* Analyses of mean plaque scores (% sites with plaque)

Results:

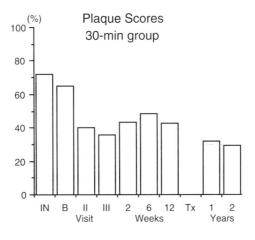

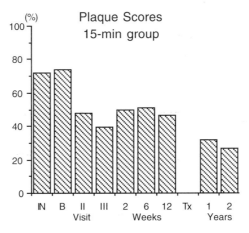

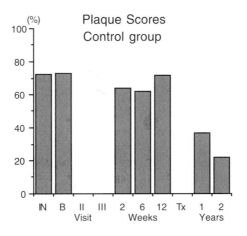

Comments:
- Similar short-term improvements of plaque scores were observed for the 30-min and 15-min groups. Thus, the effectiveness of the plaque control instruction did not seem to be influenced by the reduction of the duration of the appointments.

- The overall level for the short-term decrease of plaque scores was reached already after 1 appointment of instruction, possibly suggesting that the plaque control program could have been additionally abbreviated.

- The short-term plaque scores for the control group were minimally affected, in spite of the fact that the subjects were aware of their participation in a study.

- The plaque scores for all 3 study groups were additionally reduced during maintenance treatment.

- As compared to the white-collar subjects in the study by Söderholm et al. (1982), the plaque scores for these blue-collar workers from the same shipyard were higher, initially as well as during short-term and long-term follow-up (compare pages 255-257).

GLAVIND ET AL. (1981) compared plaque control programs which initially included a short pamphlet, a self-instructional manual or personal instruction.

Subjects and procedures:
* 37 patients, 25-64 years of age, seeking treatment at a Danish dental school

* 3 study groups matched for initial plaque scores, age and sex:
    - Pamphlet group (N=12)
    - Self-instruction group (N=12)
    - Hygienist group (N=13)

* Baseline examination followed by "scaling of the teeth"

* Procedures after 1 week:
    Pamphlet group:
    - Patients handed a short brochure on toothbrushing and on use of inter-dental woodsticks
    Self-instruction group:
    - Patients studied a self-instruction manual designed to enable them to detect insufficiently cleaned areas using plaque-disclosing dye and illuminated mouth mirror; step-wise guidance and introduction of oral hygiene aids; time for use 22-45 minutes (mean: 31 minutes)
    Hygienist group:
    - Patients instructed by a dental hygienist on a one-to-one basis; time for instruction 10-27 minutes (mean: 19 minutes)

* Patients of all 3 groups given an oral hygiene kit with toothbrush, single-tufted brush, interdental woodsticks, illuminated mouth mirror and disclosing wafers

* Procedures for all 3 groups after 2 weeks, 6 weeks and 12 weeks
    - Recording of plaque scores
    - Patients requested to clean the teeth followed by renewed scoring of plaque ("brushing test"); plaque scores used for feedback to the patients

* Recordings of presence/absence of plaque and bleeding on probing at 4 sites of each tooth (mesio-buccal, mid-buccal, disto-buccal and lingual)

* Final examination after 24 weeks

* Analyses of mean plaque and bleeding scores (% sites with plaque/bleeding)

Results:

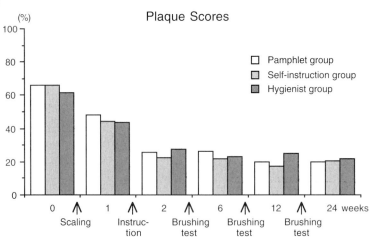

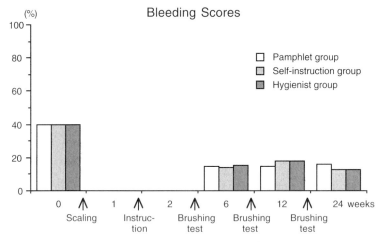

Comments:

- Plaque scores were reduced following the initial examination, which included scaling of the teeth.

- A further reduction of the plaque scores took place after oral hygiene instruction. No differences were noted relative to the mode of instruction.

- The "brushing tests" at the 2, 6 and 12-week appointments resulted in lowered plaque scores after the test as compared to before the test at all visits and for all study groups (data not shown here). Nevertheless, these tests did not seem to affect the plaque scores as recorded at the initiation of the subsequent visits. Plaque scores remained the same at 6-24 weeks as for 2 weeks.

- Bleeding on probing scores were similarly reduced for the 3 study groups. Part of the reductions may have been caused by the initial scaling of the teeth.

GLAVIND ET AL. (1985) compared self-instruction to personal instruction given by dentists.

Subjects and procedures:

* 55 patients, 20-62 years of age, from 3 general dental practices in Denmark

* 2 study groups matched for age and sex:
    - Self-instruction group (N=29)
    - Dentist group (N=26)

* Treatments:
    Self-instruction group:
    - At baseline examination: patients given a self-examination manual
    - After 1 week: patients studied a self-instruction manual and received scaling in left side of the dentition
    - After 2 weeks: plaque scores for feedback and scaling in right side of the dentition
    - After 12 weeks: plaque scores for feedback

    Dentist group:
    - At baseline examination: patients given information about oral diseases and importance of oral cleanliness by their dentist
    - After 1 week: patients provided chair-side instruction in oral hygiene by their dentist (25-30 minutes) and received scaling in left side of the dentition
    - After 2 weeks: plaque scores for feedback and scaling in right side of the dentition
    - After 12 weeks: plaque scores for feedback

* Patients of both groups given an oral hygiene kit with toothbrush, single-tufted brush, interdental woodsticks, illuminated mouth mirror and disclosing wafers

* Treatment of carious lesions as needed during the experimental period

* Recordings of presence/absence of plaque and bleeding on probing at 4 sites of each tooth (mesio-buccal, mid-buccal, disto-buccal and lingual)

* Final examination after 24 weeks

* Analyses of mean plaque and bleeding scores (% sites with plaque/bleeding)

Results:

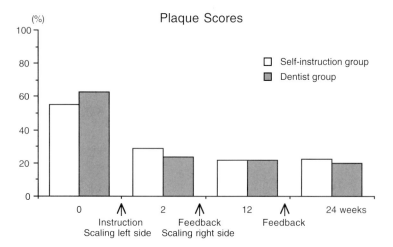

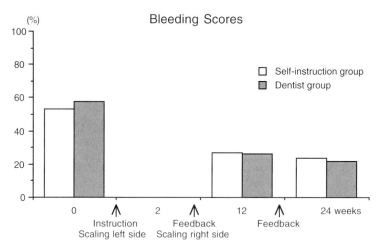

Comments:

- Similar reductions of plaque scores were observed following self-instruction and following instruction by the dentists. This confirms the findings of Glavind et al. (1981), comparing self-instruction to personal instruction by a hygienist (pages 261-262).

- Bleeding scores were also reduced to the same extent for both study groups. Part of the reductions may have been caused by the scaling of the teeth.

- Details on the distribution of patients by the 3 participating dentists and any possible differences in effectiveness of the dentists were not reported.

LIM ET AL. (1996) compared the results of oral hygiene instruction following use of self-instructional manual, video tape instruction, personal instruction and combined instructions.

Subjects and procedures:
* Originally 195 employees of a Hong Kong telephone company, 25-44 years of age

* 4 study groups :
    - Self-instruction group (original N=47)
    - Video tape instruction group (original N=46)
    - Personal instruction group (original N=54)
    - Combination instruction group (original N=48)

* No baseline prophylaxis

* Initial procedures:
    Self-instruction group:
    - Patients studied a specially designed self-instruction manual at the clinic and was given the booklet for home-use
    Video tape instruction group:
    - Patients viewed a specially designed video tape at the clinic
    Personal instruction group:
    - Patients instructed by a dental hygienist on a ono-to-one basis
    Combination instruction group:
    - Patients given a combination of 2-3 of the above modes of instruction

* Recalls after 2 and 16 weeks for demonstration of ineffectively cleaned areas; subjects having received personal instruction given renewed personal direction; other groups advised to review the respective educational material

* Recordings of presence/absence of plaque and bleeding on probing at 6 sites of each tooth

* Final examination after 40 weeks

* Analyses of mean plaque and bleeding scores (% sites with plaque/bleeding)

Results:

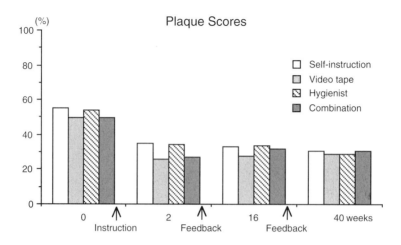

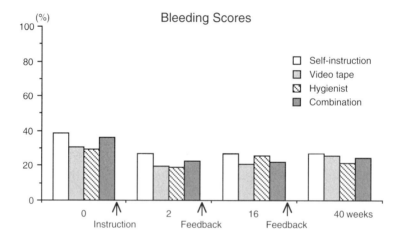

Comments:

- Plaque scores were reduced similarly for the 4 different groups following the initial instruction.

- The reinforcements after 2 and 16 weeks did not result in any further reduction of the plaque scores.

- Bleeding scores were modestly affected in all 4 groups.

- The authors remarked on "the omnipresence of calculus in the participants". This may have limited the impact on both plaque and bleeding scores.

- Overall, 12% of the subjects did not complete the study.

TEDESCO ET AL. (1992) studied the effects of additional feedback using microscopic demonstrations of the patients' own subgingival microflora.

Subjects and procedures:

* Originally 167 subjects, 21-65 years of age, recruited for study in a city in USA by announcements in local media

* 2 study groups:
  - Experimental group (original N=111)
  - Control group (original N=56)

* Baseline examination followed by prophylaxis

* Oral hygiene instruction and a 2nd prophylaxis 1 month later, followed by 3 monthly visits for feedback

* Procedures:
  Control group:
  - At the 1-month visit, patients received information on their oral health and instructions in brushing and flossing techniques by a dental hygien-ist, followed by a 2nd prophylaxis; at the 2-, 3- and 4-month visits patients received feedback on which teeth and surfaces needed most improvement
  Experimental group:
  - In addition to the treatment given to the control group, patients were shown a phase contrast slide of their own subgingival microflora on a video monitor; at the 1-month visit both before and after prophylaxis emphasizing the difference; at the 2-, 3- and 4-month visits with com-parison to the video demonstration from previous visit and relating the microscopic results to the plaque and gingivitis scores

* Plaque scores at 4 locations of each tooth using Silness-Löe index (scores 0-3)

* Gingivitis scores at 4 locations of each tooth using Löe-Silness index (scores 0-3)

* Final examination after 13 months

* Analyses of mean plaque and gingivitis scores

Results:

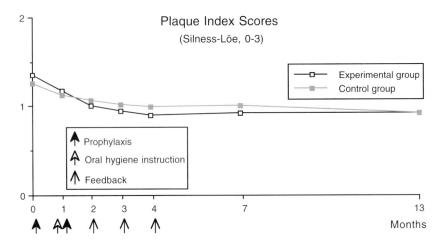

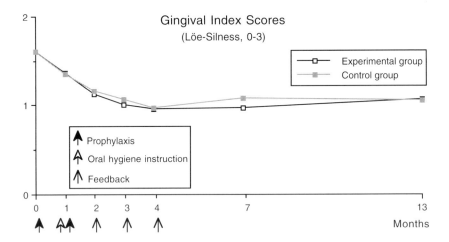

Comments:

- Plaque scores were similarly and modestly reduced for both study groups.

- Gingivitis scores also decreased to the same extent for both groups. These reductions may to some extent be explained by the prophylaxes given at baseline and 1 month.

- This study suffered from a high dropout rate. Only 52% of control subjects and 55% of experimental subjects completed the study. The authors did not offer any explanation for this.

Oral hygiene instruction

Concluding remarks

Plaque control instruction may result in significant short-term improvement of oral hygiene as evaluated from reductions of plaque and bleeding scores. Average plaque scores for the entire dentition of untreated groups of patients amounting to 65-75% can be reduced to levels of 15-30%. Long-term follow-ups of patients on regular recalls have shown that it is possible to maintain the initial improvements.

The mode of instruction may not be critical. However, the subjects participating in the studies have been examined at repeated intervals and are aware that their plaque scores will be evaluated. It seems difficult to separate the influence of these repeated examinations from the effects of the instructions. This limitation of study design may partly explain why studies so far have failed to identify factors of importance for effective oral hygiene instruction. The relevance of the experimental studies, therefore, may be questioned.

Results of studies on plaque control instruction given to groups of patients indicate a relationship between pre- and postinstruction scores, i.e. individuals with higher scores before instruction tend to show higher scores also after instruction, and vice versa. Apart from this, studies have failed to find associations between various patient characteristics and outcome of oral hygiene instruction (Ödman et al. 1984, Glavind 1986). In other words, we do not know why some individuals are more easily motivated than others. There is neither any knowledge why some therapists may be more effective than others. Thus, the answer to the question about the key to successful plaque control instruction can not be based upon results of studies. The answer will need to be speculative and based upon the presence of a possible common denominator in the available studies showing successful results: Create an atmosphere of utmost importance with respect to plaque control.

The available studies - those reviewed here and others - have focused on short-term evaluations. It is not known when a relapse towards baseline values should be anticipated. However, lack of recall and lack of continued emphasis on proper oral hygiene eventually appear to result in regression (e.g. Axelsson & Lindhe 1981a, 1981b).

Oral hygiene instruction

References

Axelsson, P. & Lindhe, J. (1981a) Effect of controlled oral hygiene procedures on caries and periodontal disease in adults. Results after 6 years. Journal of Clinical Periodontology 8, 239-248.

Axelsson, P. & Lindhe, J. (1981b) The significance of maintenance care in the treatment of periodontal disease. Journal of Clinical Periodontology 8, 281-294.

Glavind, L. (1986) The result of periodontal treatment in relation to various background factors. Journal of Clinical Periodontology 13, 789-794.

Glavind, L., Zeuner, E. & Attström, R. (1981) Oral hygiene instruction of adults by means of a self-instructional manual. Journal of Clinical Periodontology 8, 165-176.

Glavind, L., Christensen, H., Pedersen, E., Rosendahl, H. & Attström, R. (1985) Oral hygiene instruction in general dental practice by means of self-teaching manuals. Journal of Clinical Periodontology 12, 27-34.

Lim, L.P., Davies, W.I.R., Yuen, K.W. & Ma, M.H. (1996) Comparison of modes of oral hygiene instruction in improving gingival health. Journal of Clinical Periodontology 23, 693-697.

Söderholm, G. & Egelberg, J. (1982) Teaching plaque control. II. 30-minute versus 15-minute appointments in a three-visit program. Journal of Clinical Periodontology 9, 214-222.

Söderholm, G., Nobréus, N., Attström, R. & Egelberg, J. (1982) Teaching plaque control. I. A five-visit versus a two-visit program. Journal of Clinical Periodontology 9, 203-213.

Tedesco, L.A., Keffer, M.A., Davis, E.L. & Christersson, L.A. (1992) Effect of a social cognitive intervention on oral health status, behavior reports, and cognitions. Journal of Periodontology 63, 567-575.

Ödman, P.A., Lange, A.L. & Bakdash, B. (1984) Utilization of locus of control in the prediction of patients' oral hygiene performance. Journal of Clinical Periodontology 11, 367-372.

APPENDIX 1

Commonly used plaque and gingival indices

Turesky/Quigley-Hein Plaque Index
Following use of disclosing dye, buccal and lingual aspects of the teeth are scored for presence of plaque as follows:

0 = No plaque.

1 = Separate flecks of plaque at the cervical margin of the tooth.

2 = A thin continuous band of plaque (up to 1 mm) at the cervical margin.

3 = A band of plaque wider than 1 mm but covering less than 1/3 of the crown.

4 = Plaque covering at least 1/3 but less than 2/3 of the crown.

5 = Plaque covering 2/3 or more of the crown.

This index records the extension of plaque over the tooth surface. Use of disclosing dye means that a score of 0 and also a score of 1 may be difficult to reach by many patients, since a thin film of deposits will result in a positive score. A score of 5 is probably uncommon for teeth in normal alignment, since friction from cheeks, lips, tongue and food tends to keep the coronal parts of the crowns free from plaque. A score of 4 may also be uncommon, at least for people who use a toothbrush on a daily basis.

According to the Turesky et al. (1970) modification of the original index by Quigley & Hein (1962), a score should be given for each of buccal and lingual aspects of the teeth. Later, however, investigators have often given separate scores for 6 aspects of each tooth (mesio-buccal, mid-buccal, disto-buccal, mesio-lingual, mid-lingual and disto-lingual).

Silness-Löe Plaque Index

As described by Löe (1967), the teeth are scored for the presence of plaque without the use of disclosing dye as follows:

0 = The gingival area of the tooth surface is literally free of plaque. The surface is tested by running a pointed probe across the tooth surface at the entrance of the gingival crevice after the tooth has been properly dried. If no soft matter adheres to the point of the probe, the area is considered clean.

1 = No plaque can be observed in situ by the unaided eye, but the plaque is made visible on the point of the probe after it has been moved across the tooth surface at the entrance of the gingival crevice.

2 = The gingival area is covered with a thin to moderately thick layer of plaque. The deposit is visible to the naked eye.

3 = Heavy accumulation of soft matter, the thickness of which fills out the niche produced by the gingival margin and the tooth surface. The inter-dental area is stuffed with soft debris.

This index focuses on the amounts of plaque at the gingival margin. It was introduced since it may be more related to risk for development of caries and periodontal disease than an index like Turesky/Quigley-Hein which records the extension of plaque over the tooth surface.

A score of 0 for Silness-Löe index is less demanding than a 0 score for the Turesky/Quigley-Hein index. A Silness-Löe score of 3 may not be uncommon in careless brushers.

Originally, as described by Silness & Löe (1964), separate scores should be given for 4 aspects of each tooth (mesial, buccal, distal, lingual). Some investigators have examined mesial and distal surfaces from the buccal aspect only, while others have inspected mesial and distal surfaces from both buccal and lingual aspects and recorded the highest score. Separate records from 6 aspects of each tooth, however, are commonly used (mesio-buccal, mid-buccal, disto-buccal, mesio-lingual, mid-lingual and disto-lingual).

% Sites with Plaque

Presence or absence of plaque at the gingival margin is recorded. Plaque scores are expressed as % of examined sites showing plaque. Records may be taken:
- following use of a disclosing dye;
- using the tip of a probe moved along the gingival margin to make the plaque discernible; or
- using the unaided eye ('visible plaque').

Presence/absence scores may be an advantage to graded plaque indices, since the degree of subjectivity during scoring is reduced. On the other hand, dichotomized presence/absence scores do not allow determination of degrees of plaque accumulation at the individual site. Some investigators have obtained records using a graded index, and then presented their findings both using the graded index and using presence/absence scores (positive scores of the graded index versus zero scores; % sites with positive scores of examined sites).

Rustogi/Navy Plaque Index

During recording, the examiner identifies a total of 9 different locations of each buccal and lingual surface. Presence/absence of plaque is scored following use of a disclosing dye for each of these sites:
- 3 narrow zones along the gingival margin (mesial, middle and distal);
- 2 narrow proximal zones (mesial and distal; adjacent to the tip of the interdental papillae); and
- 4 sites on the remaining tooth surface (1 apical, 2 middle and 1 coronal).

This index was introduced to allow for more detailed analyses along the gingival margin and for proximal sites. Results may be expressed as % of examined sites showing plaque:
- for gingival margin sites;
- for proximal sites; and
- for all sites.

This index, thus requires that the examiner scores as many as 18 different sites per tooth, and that the examiner is sufficiently trained to be able to identify and separate the various sites in a consistent manner throughout the dentition. This exacting task may explain why this index has been used less frequently than others.

Löe-Silness Gingival Index

The severity of gingival inflammation is recorded as follows:

0 = Absence of inflammation.

1 = Mild inflammation; slight change in color and little change in texture.

2 = Moderate inflammation; moderate glazing, redness, edema and hyper-trophy; bleeding on pressure.

3 = Severe inflammation; marked redness and hypertrophy; tendency to spontaneous bleeding; ulceration.

Over the years, investigators seem to have 'modified' the application of score 2 of this index and primarily considered the bleeding aspect, as recorded after passing a periodontal probe along the inside of the gingival crevice using a light force.

Originally, as described by Löe & Silness (1963), separate scores should be given for 4 aspects of each tooth (mesial, buccal, distal, lingual). Some investigators have examined mesial and distal surfaces from the buccal aspect only, while others have inspected mesial and distal surfaces from both buccal and lingual aspects and recorded the highest score. Separate records from 6 aspects of each tooth, however, are commonly used (mesio-buccal, mid-buccal, disto-buccal, mesio-lingual, mid-lingual and disto-lingual).

Lobene Gingival Index

The severity of gingival inflammation is recorded from the buccal and lingual aspects of each tooth as follows:

0 = Absence of inflammation.

1 = Mild inflammation; slight change in color, little change in texture of any portion of, but not the entire marginal or papillary gingival unit.

2 = Moderate inflammation; criteria as above but involving the entire marginal or papillary gingival unit.

3 = Severe inflammation; glazing, redness, edema and/or hypertrophy of the marginal or papillary gingival unit.

4 = Severe inflammation; marked redness, edema and/or hypertrophy of the marginal or papillary gingival unit, spontaneous bleeding, congestion or ulceration.

This index is a modification of the Löe-Silness index and was introduced by Lobene et al. (1986) for the purpose of providing an increased sensitivity in the lower degree of inflammation and to eliminate the bleeding on pressure component. Since bleeding is not a criterion, intra- and interexaminer calibrations and reproducibility test can be performed at the same patient visit.

Marginal and papillary units are scored separately for each of the buccal and lingual aspects of the teeth.

% Sites with Gingivitis

Some investigators, after obtaining records using Löe-Silness or Lobene gingival index, have presented the results both using the graded index and presence/absence scores (positive scores of the graded index versus zero scores; % sites with positive scores of examined sites).

Bleeding on Probing

Presence or absence of bleeding following probing (as for probing depth measurement) is recorded and expressed as % bleeding sites out of all examined sites in the dentition.

Bleeding on probing may relate more closely to the level of chronic inflammation in the gingival tissue than the more superficial signs of redness, glazing and edema. In addition, the degree of subjectivity during scoring is reduced, especially if probing is performed with a standardized probing force using a pressure sensitive probe. On the other hand, dichotomized presence/absence scores do not allow determination of degrees in 'inflammation' at the individual site. Some investigators have applied and analyzed their data using both a gingival index and bleeding on probing scores.

Bleeding indices have been developed which assign numerical values to the quickness of bleeding and/or the extent of bleeding following probing. These indices have not been commonly used, presumably due to the drawbacks of using such numerical index scores.

Eastman Interdental Bleeding Index

A dichotomous scoring system with presence or absence of interdental bleeding following 4 x interdental insertion and papillary depression with a triangular woodstick was introduced by Caton & Polson (1985). The % bleeding interdental areas in the dentition is calculated. This method has primarily been used in studies focusing on interdental cleaning and gingivitis control.

Commonly used plaque and gingival indices

Concluding remarks

Plaque and gingival indices have been introduced since degrees of plaque accumulation and levels of gingivitis can not easily be determined with objective measurements. Increasing degrees of plaque/gingivitis are given increasing numerical values as described for the various indices.

Some of the limitations of these index systems should be recognized:

- Due to the subjective nature of the scoring systems, investigators may vary in their application of the verbal descriptions of the scores. In addition, the same examiner may change his/her application over time, e.g. during the course of a study (see 'examiner calibration' and 'examiner drift' in Appendix 2: Glossary of Experimental Designs, pages 279-291).

- The numerical scores do not represent a mathematical continuous scale, i.e. an index score of 2 is not necessarily twice as much as an index score of 1, an index score of 3 is not 3 times as much as an index score of 1, etc. This means that averages should not be calculated and evaluated statistically. Although averages could be calculated and used for overall descriptive purposes, statistics should be based upon frequency distributions of the various scores, i.e. experimental groups should be compared with respect to the frequency of occurrence of the various score levels. In spite of the fact that this has long been recognized, most investigators continue to base their statistics on averages of scores.

- Plaque and gingivitis scores for proximal sites in individuals with intact interdental papillary heights represent the visible part of the proximal locations and not the region located under the contact points between the teeth. Plaque and gingivitis in this latter location, often termed interdental, most likely relate more to development of caries and periodontitis, but can not be detected and recorded unless the papillary height has been reduced. The difference between proximal and interdental locations should be kept in mind while interpreting the clinical studies.

Commonly used plaque and gingival indices

References

Caton, J.G. & Polson, A.M. (1985) The interdental bleeding index: a simplified procedure for monitoring gingival health. Compendium of Continuing Education in Dentistry 6, 88-92.

Lobene, R.R., Weatherford, T., Ross, N.M., Lamm, R.A. & Menaker, L. (1986) A modified gingival index for use in clinical trials. Clinical Preventive Dentistry 8 (I), 3-6.

Löe, H. (1967) The gingival index, the plaque index and the retention index systems. Journal of Periodontology 38, 610-616.

Löe, H. & Silness, J. (1963) Periodontal disease in pregnancy. (I). Prevalence and severity, Acta Odontologica Scandinavia 21, 533-551.

Quigley, G.A. & Hein, J.W. (1962) Comparative cleansing efficiency of manual and power brushing. Journal of the American Dental Association 65, 26-29.

Rustogi, K.N., Curtis, J.P., Volpe, A.R., Kemp, J.H., McCool, J.J. & Korn, L.R. (1992) Refinement of the modified navy plaque index to increase plaque scoring efficiency in gumline and interproximal tooth areas. Journal of Clinical Dentistry, 3, suppl C, C9-C12.

Silness, J. & Löe, H. (1964) Periodontal disease in pregnancy. (II). Correlation between oral hygiene and periodontal condition. Acta Odontologica Scandinavia 22, 121-135.

Turesky, S., Gilmore, N.D. & Glickman, I. (1970) Reduced plaque formation by the chloromethyl analogue of victamine C. Journal of Periodontology 41, 41-43.

Glossary of experimental designs

Alternating sequence   See cross-over design.

Balanced groups   See parallel design.

Baseline examination   Baseline examination is undertaken at the start of a study. A *screening examination* of subjects volunteering for a study may be required prior to baseline for the purpose of selecting subjects meeting determined inclusion and exclusion criteria. The term *initial examination* is less specific and is sometimes used for screening examination and sometimes for baseline examination.

Baseline prophylaxis   In studies on oral hygiene methods, a baseline with teeth free from dental plaque and calculus is often desirable. The teeth are professionally cleaned to achieve plaque score = 0.

Baseline prophylaxis is less suited in studies with emphasis on gingivitis effects. The prophylaxis may have a significant gingivitis reducing effect, confounding possible gingivitis effects of the investigated procedures. In addition, the potential for finding difference between various experimental procedures may become reduced.

Some trials have used baseline prophylaxis for half of the dentition only (diagonal quadrants). This design provides an evaluation of the procedures under study with and without prior prophylaxis.

Carry-over effect   See cross-over design.

Clinical importance   See statistical significance.

Clinical significance   See statistical significance.

Coded records   Examination records for the various study groups are given codes instead of being labelled with actual test procedure. The codes are not broken until completion of data analysis. This eliminates the impact of any investigator bias during conduct of study and during analysis of results.

Compliance   Compliance to the experimental procedures by participating subjects is often critical. Example: a long-term study evaluating the effects of mouthrinses to supplement mechanical plaque control would be of little value without proper compliance. Investigators often use a combination of measures to maintain compliance. Subjects may be asked to report back to the clinic with regular intervals, e.g. every 2 weeks. At these occasions they return the bottle of mouthwash apportioned for the latest 2 weeks in exchange for a new bottle. In addition, they hand in completed daily rinsing records for the same period in exchange for a new diary form. These procedures may be combined with an emphasis on honesty of reports ('everybody may forget, but please let us know if/when you do').

Comparative study   See controlled study.

Control group   See controlled study.

Controlled study   A controlled study has *experimental* or *test* groups and a *control group*, i.e. the experimental procedure or procedures are compared to no treatment. In studies on drugs, the test drugs are often compared to use of a *placebo* (= *vehicle control*; vehicle only, no active ingredients).

In a *comparative study*, 2 or more experimental procedures are compared without the inclusion of a control group. A control group may not always be necessary and may sometimes be unethical. Example: studies on effectiveness of novel design toothbrushes need to be comparative.

Cross-over design

With this experimental design, the same group of subjects are exposed to both experimental and control procedures. Example: 20 subjects have been recruited for a 3-week study on a mouthrinse. The subjects are first devided into 2 groups of 10 subjects each. One of these groups starts using the mouthrinse and the other group starts using the placebo rinse during the first 3-week period. After an interval with regular oral hygiene without any rinse (*wash-out period*), the use of mouthrinse and placebo is switched between the groups for a 2nd 3-week period. A wash-out period is needed since the procedure during the 1st 3-week interval may have resulted in some change that does not disappear once rinsing is discontinued. Such a residual condition could affect the outcome of the 2nd 3-week period (*carry-over effect*).

Should 3 experimental/control procedures be evaluated, recruited subjects are devided into 3 groups, followed by use of 3 experimental periods, separated by wash-out periods. The turn of use of the 3 procedures are arranged to allow each procedure being used during each of the 3 experimental periods (*alternating/ rotating sequence*). An example using 3 groups/procedures (A, B and C) is given below:

Period	Groups		
1	A	B	C
2	B	C	A
3	C	A	B

Cross-over designs for 4 or more procedures are constructed in a similar manner.

Dental prophylaxis   See baseline prophylaxis.

Double-blind design   See single-blind design.

Examiner calibration   An examiner using a recording system like a plaque index is expected to translate written descriptions of the criteria for the index scores into the clinical situation. Interpretations may vary among examiners. A certain amount of variation in these applications will always take place, but needs to be kept to a minimum. In examiner calibration, examiners conduct practice sessions and compare and harmonize their recordings. After such training sessions, the examiners evaluate the degree of reproducibility of their recordings. The same group of patients is examined separately by 2 examiners and their results compared (*interexaminer reproducibility*). Also, the same examiner may examine the same patients at 2 separate occasions and compare the results (*intraexaminer reproducibility*).

Acceptable levels of reproducibility is critical for the possibility of discovering differences between experimental procedures. Inconsistency of recordings will reduce the possibility of finding true differences. If a study finds no difference between procedures, this may be related to inconsistent examiner recordings.

In studies with many subjects, 2 or more examiners may be used, each examining the same individuals throughout the study. This arrangement may be required for practical reasons, but increases the need for proper examiner calibration and acceptable interexaminer reproducibility. Naturally, examiner calibration is an important part of preparation for multicenter studies, where geographical reasons often require a different examiner at each study location.

Examiner drift   Using subjective scoring systems like plaque and gingival indices, an examiner may change the implementation of the scoring system somewhat over time.

Awareness of the phenomenon of examiner drift is particularly important in long-term parallel design studies. Repeated calibrations and determinations of interexaminer reproducibility to other experienced clinicians during the course of the study can be used to minimize the potential for examiner drift.

Exclusion criteria See inclusion criteria.

Experimental effect See Hawthorne effect.

Experimental group See controlled study.

Hawthorne effect Participation in a study makes the subjects aware and attentive to the particular conditions under study. Example: subjects in a study comparing different toothbrushes may brush their teeth more carefully than normally. This *experimental* or *participation effect* is a well-known phenomenon and may confound the interpretation of results (first described in a study at a factory in Hawthorne, IL, USA).

Informed consent According to international rules, any participation in a study must to be on a volunteer basis, and also following reviewing written information about the nature of the trial. Volunteers leave their consent by signing the information document, which also states that the subjects have the right to withdraw from the study at any time.

Inclusion criteria Sets of inclusion criteria and *exclusion criteria* are used to define individuals qualifying as study subjects.

Initial examination See baseline examination.

Matched groups See parallel design.

Multicenter study Subjects are recruited at different locations. At each of these sites, the same study procedures are duplicated.

This arrangement may be necessary to enable recruitment of sufficient number of subjects, e.g. to allow an evaluation of the incidence of possible side effects. A multicenter approach may also be selected for the purpose of assessing the reliability of the findings, i.e. to find out if there are any variations in outcome when the same procedures are conducted among different people. Most often, multicenter studies use different examiners at the various locations, which calls for calibration of these examiners (see examiner calibration).

Novelty effect

Subjects introduced to a new method of plaque control (e.g. the use of a novel design electric toothbrush) may be more attentive and thorough using this method during an initial period of time than the familiar use of a conventional product. This will favor the results for the new product. Long-term studies are required to reduce the possibility of such novelty effect.

Outcome variable

See parameter.

Overnight plaque

In studies on oral hygiene methods, subjects are often instructed not to use any hygiene procedures on the day of examination prior to the recordings. This system may reduce the subjects' tendency to make an extra effort prior to the examinations, thereby providing more representative plaque scores.

Parameter

A measurement like plaque index and gingival index recorded to determine study outcome (*outcome variable*).

Parallel design

With this experimental design, recruited subjects are devided into experimental/control groups and carried through the study in parallel during one study period only.

With this design, some procedure should be used to assure that the subjects in the various groups are comparable at the onset of the study (*balanced groups*).

For example, a study comparing effects of various toothbrush designs on plaque and gingivitis needs comparable study groups with respect to baseline plaque and gingivitis scores, and maybe also with respect to other factors like age, sex and number of remaining teeth.

Accomplishment of balanced groups starts with the use of narrow criteria for recruitment of subjects into the study. Example: only subjects between 30-50 years, having a full dentition without evidence of destructive periodontal disease, having full mouth Quigley-Hein plaque scores ≥ 2 and full mouth bleeding scores $\geq 50\%$. The recruited subjects will then be *randomly distributed* (*randomly allocated*) among the study groups using a random system (e.g. random tables). With sufficient number of subjects, such procedures will probably result in adequately balanced groups.

To guarantee balanced study groups with respect to certain criteria, a different approached may be used. Based on the results of a screening examination, all participants are ranked with respect to a given criterion, e.g. bleeding scores. Should 3 study groups be needed, those 3 individuals having the highest bleeding scores of all subjects (ranks 1, 2 and 3) are first separated into 3 groups using a random system. Subsequently, individuals with ranks 4, 5 and 6 are randomly distributed into the 3 groups, etc., until all subjects have been assigned their groups. In this way, *matched groups* are formed with respect to a given criterion. It is also possible and more common to match groups with respect to several criteria. For this matching, the various criteria could be given different weight or priority. The formation of matched groups is often termed *stratification*.

Participation effect   See Hawthorne effect.

Placebo group   See controlled study.

Placebo effect   In studies on drugs, test drugs are often compared to use of a *placebo* (= *vehicle control*; vehicle only, no active ingredients). Some improvements, e.g. reductions of pain, are commonly observed for subjects belonging to placebo groups. This is believed to be a psychological/physiological reaction caused by the anticipation that a drug has treatment effects and a desire to obtain relief of symptoms, possibly coupled with a will to please the therapist. Thus, an inactivated placebo drug is perceived to have some treatment effect. Example: treatment of dentine hypersensitivity.

Publication bias   Researchers are looking for discoveries and innovations. In a field like oral hygiene methods, investigators are often evaluating new products which potentially may be improvements over previous ones. Positive findings will most likely be published. Negative findings may not reach the literature. This means that a review of the available literature may not reflect the true status of the total research that has been carried out about a given method. Example: let us assume that 3 similar studies have been undertaken on the effectiveness of a particular powered toothbrush. In 2 of these trials, the powered brush was found to be somewhat superior to manual toothbrushing. In the 3rd study, the results showed no difference between powered and manual brushing. There is a possibility that only the 2 studies with positive results reached the literature. If so, the reader will be biased by what has been published.

Quadrate design   See split-mouth design.

Ramfjord teeth   In order to reduce the number of teeth to be recorded, 6 teeth are selected which are considered representative for the entire dentition (as suggested by Ramfjord): right maxillary 1st premolar, left maxillary 1st incisor, left maxillary 1st molar, right mandibular 1st molar, right mandibular 1st incisor and left mandibular 1st premolar.

Random allocation	See parallel design.
Random distribution	See parallel design.
Reproducibility	See examiner calibration.
Rotating sequence	See cross-over design.
Sample size	See subjects.
Screening examination	See baseline examination.

Single-blind design

The examiner is unaware ('blinded') of group assignment for individual subjects in order to conduct unbiased examinations. This is a basic requirement for experimental trials.

Whenever possible, the subjects should also be 'blinded' to the procedure they are exposed to. Example: subjects in control groups of mouthrinse studies are given the 'same' mouthrinse, bottled similarly, with all ingredients (solvents, flavors etc.) except the active agent (= placebo). A *double-blind design* has both examiners and subjects 'blinded' to the procedures.

Due to obvious reasons, studies on toothbrushes and interdental aids can only have a single-blind design. Trials on dentifrices and mouthrinses, however, should have a double-blind design.

Split-mouth design

Experimental conditions/procedures are varied in left and right halves of the dentition (or between diagonal pairs of quadrants). Example: the effect of a mouthrinse may want to be studied having professionally cleaned teeth for baseline (plaque scores = 0), but also without baseline prophylaxis. A spilt-mouth design using prophylaxis in half of the dentition can be used.

Experimental procedures may also be varied between all 4 quadrants of the dentition (*quadrant design*).

Statistical significance Various types of statistical tests need to be used for the analyses of results in order to find out if seeming differences between procedures are real. A difference between procedures reaching statistical significance means that such a difference is probably not due to chance. This does not mean, however, that this difference has *clinical significance* or *clinical importance*. Example: use of a mouthrinse during 3 weeks without mechanical plaque control has resulted in a mean Silness-Löe plaque index score of 1.6 for the mouthrinse group as compared to 2.0 for the placebo group. This means that the mouthrinse has reduced plaque formation by 20%, a difference that most likely will show statistical significance if reasonably large study groups are used. We may, however, consider this difference without clinical relevance, since a plaque score of 1.6 may have a similar disease potential as a score of 2.0.

In this context, it should be pointed out that the reader of any study on oral hygiene methods showing difference in plaque and gingivitis scores between procedures should ask himself/herself to what extent the difference observed may have some impact on caries and periodontal disease progression. In fact, herein lies one of the major difficulties in evaluation of oral hygiene studies.

Stratification See parallel design.

Study groups See subjects.

Subjects Subjects recruited for a trial should fulfil 2 basic requirements: 1) they should be suited for participation relative to the purpose of the study (appropriate *study groups*); 2) they should be sufficiently many to provide reliable findings (adequate *sample size* to provide sufficiently large study groups) .

1) Appropriate study groups:
Example: a study investigating the effectiveness of a novel design manual toothbrush should include subjects with gingivitis, but without any reduction of the interdental papillary heights. It is not to be expected that use of a manual brush would provide any significant interdental cleaning. Inclusion of subjects with reduced papillary heights, therefore, might mask an advantage to the new design brush that would have been observed had only intact dentitions been included. (Presence of occasional interdental areas with reduced papillae - or diastema between the teeth - can be handled by exclusion of these areas from study.)

Also, subjects included in a manual toothbrush study should not exhibit periodontal pockets ≥ 4 mm deep, since supragingival plaque control has limited potentials to affect gingival inflammation in such areas. (Again, presence of occasional pockets ≥ 4 mm can be handled by exclusion of these areas from study.)

Obviously, any characteristic which may make a subject unsuited for inclusion in a particular study needs to be considered.

2) Sufficiently large study groups:
From a statistical perspective, results from a trial are only absolutely true for the very subjects that were included in the study, unless the subjects represent a random sample of an entire population. Subjects for studies on oral hygiene methods are seldom such random samples due to the efforts required for such recruitment. This means, however, that generalization of findings to other individuals should actually not be made. Nevertheless, investigators generally make clinical recommendations based upon their findings from nonrandom samples. Empirically, it appears that this 'tradition' is acceptable.

The issue of size of study groups becomes a matter of judgement. Is it reasonable to make clinical recommendations from a study having this particular number of individuals of this specific character? How large is the possibility that positive findings in favor of a given procedure (with statistical significance) in a trial with few individuals may only be valid for the subjects under study? How large is the possibility that negative findings - no difference between procedures - may be due to an unusually great variation in response to the procedures in a study with limited number of subjects (reducing the power of the statistical tests).

Investigators on oral hygiene methods using parallel design (study groups with different subjects) have most often used groups of 30 or more individuals, although studies with about 20 subjects per group are also available. Trials using cross-over design (same subjects) commonly include fewer individuals than the parallel design studies, often around 20 subjects.

Although the above numbers seem low, matters of practicability and expense need to be considered. To be accepted as the 'truth', the results of a single study on a particular question ought to be verified, irrespective of the sample size, by one or more additional studies performed by other investigators. Acceptance of somewhat limited sample sizes may be necessary and to be preferred in order to increase the likelihood of obtaining such verification.

Supervised procedures Supervised procedures are used to reduce or eliminate the risk of poor compliance. Example: in studies on mouthrinses, subjects may be visiting the clinic during week-days for supervised rinsings.

Test group See controlled study.

Validity   A given measurement used in a study may be more or less valid depending upon how well it reflects the overall intent. Example: use of a plaque index system that reflects the extension of plaque over buccal and lingual surfaces may have limited validity if our main interests focus on caries and periodontal disease. A plaque index recording the amounts of plaque along the gingival margin, particularly for proximal surfaces may be more valid.

Vehicle control   See controlled study.

Wash-out period   See cross-over design.